REVISED AND
EXPANDED EDITION

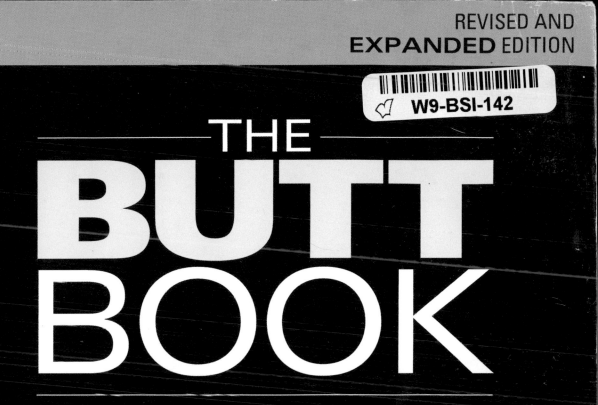

THE
BUTT
BOOK

How to Build a
Non-Cellulite & Fat-Free Butt in
9 Weeks!

TOSCARENO
B.Sc., B.Ed.

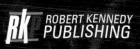 ROBERT KENNEDY
PUBLISHING

Published by Robert Kennedy Publishing
5775 McLaughlin Road
Mississauga, ON
L5R 3P7 Canada

Design by Gabriella Caruso Marques
Edited by Wendy Morley

National Library of Canada Cataloguing in Publication

Reno, Tosca, 1959-
        The Butt Book : How to build a non-cellulite and fat free butt in 9 weeks! /
Tosca Reno.--Rev. and expanded ed.

ISBN-13: 978-1-55210-041-7
ISBN-10: 1-55210-041-3

        1. Buttocks exercises. 2. Exercise for women. 3. Buttocks
 I. Title.

GV508.R45 2007   613.7'1888   C2007-901328-7

10 9 8 7 6 5 4 3 2 1

Distributed in Canada by
National Book Network
67 Mowat Avenue, Suite 241
Toronto, ON
M6K 3E3

Distributed in USA by
National Book Network
15200 NBN Way
Blue Ridge Sumitt, PA
17214

Printed in Canada

contents

foreword

Is your job making your butt fat? Do you absolutely hate walking ahead of someone in the hallway or up a flight of stairs, fearing that they are checking out your rear at every step?

Most women throw the blame for their less-than-perfect butts on the fact that women's glutes carry added fat necessary for child bearing, or that they have to log too many hours at work in their office chairs. Of course there's always the genetic factor to blame, or the fact that as children they were fed too many calories ...

Whatever the current condition of your butt, it can be changed. I promise you it can be changed! Simply follow author Tosca Reno's advice and you will get there. Tosca herself weighed over 200 pounds and changed her body – and her butt – to bring it to the gorgeous shape it's in today. Don't let anyone tell you that you can't get an amazing backside. Yes, you do have to be motivated, and yes, it takes effort and dedication. But give this book a chance, follow the steps and you will know a joy that you haven't experienced in years! Good luck. Your bootylicious days are ahead.

Robert Kennedy,
Publisher, *Oxygen* Magazine

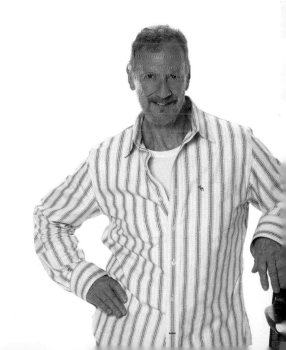

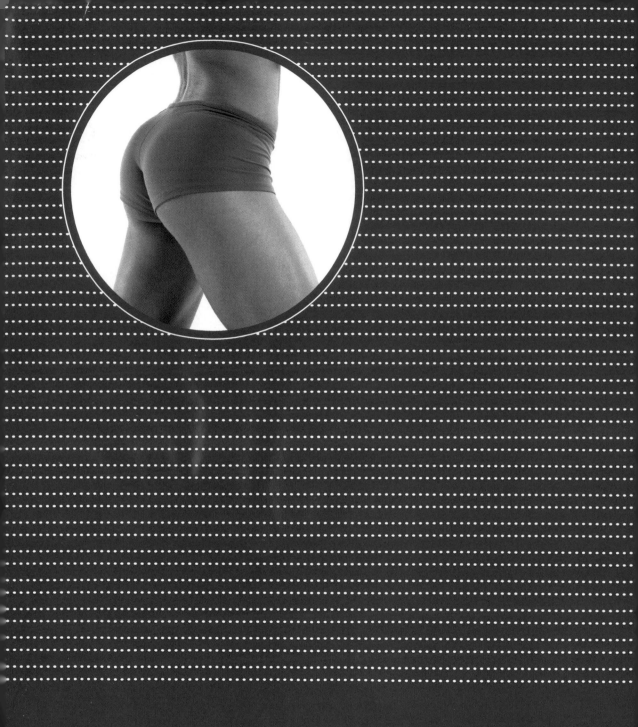

butt basics 101

what does a beautiful
backside **look like?**

What has dimples, cheeks and a crack and comes in the form of apples, pears or watermelons? You don't have to look far for the answer; you're probably sitting on it. It's your gluteus maximus, the largest of the 639 named muscles in the human body. Compared to animals, humans have rather large posteriors because we walk on two legs, which support all of our body weight, while animals have four legs to support their weight.

While your posterior may be out of your view, it is on display for everyone else to see. No doubt you've noticed how different everyone's hind quarters are. Some are flat and skinny while others are fat, bulging and jiggly, hence the comparison to fruit. It is the very rare rear indeed that is toned and perky like a granny smith apple.

what are the glutes?

The glutes are pure muscle, each cheek weighing on average one kilogram. The glutes are the workhorses of the body, allowing us to perform a multitude of functions from running to walking to dancing. We may think the buttocks are just one giant muscle but there are three muscle groups in the hip region, each one qualified by size. The gluteus maximus is the largest muscle and gives the buttock area its familiar shape. The gluteus medius is the middle-sized muscle and the gluteus minimus is the smallest. The gluteus maximus extends the thigh while the other gluteal muscles work in concert to keep the pelvis level and to swing the opposite leg forward while walking.

muscle or not?

North Americans are particularly uptight about the buttocks because most do not consider the glutes to be a muscle group. This may result from the fact that many butts are in no way muscular – too many doughnuts, chips and pies will do that to a person's posterior. Many think that butt is a dirty four-letter word simply because the posterior hides our more intimate places. This is narrow-minded thinking. The biceps too are muscles but are not considered to

"Strong glutes will help support the core, decrease risk of injury, improve posture and, of course, look great in a bikini."

be sexually offensive. Indeed, a well-toned backside can be most appealing in the same way that any well-toned muscle is appealing simply because it represents all that is robust and alive in a vital person. When you see a saggy backside you get the feeling that you are looking at someone who is fundamentally unfit, unwell and lazy – a misconception born out of the notion that fat people have some sort of "fat disease."

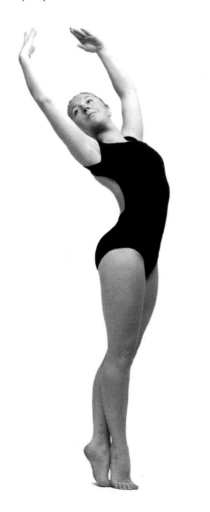

A tight pair of glutes is a glorious sight and speaks of the enormous amount of self-discipline required to eat and exercise correctly on a daily basis. It is in no way offensive to watch a gymnast muscle her way gracefully through a floor routine, her tight little buttocks propelling her forward. Nor is it off-putting to witness the balletic performance of a prima ballerina whose body is so tight and lean that her exquisite lines make you want to cry. The same cannot be said of a giant hind end that can hardly walk let alone sit down, as the flesh hangs dangerously down, burgeoning with the weight of pounds of deadly fat.

does my butt look like that?

I recall lying on a sunny beach in the Caribbean not long ago. A heavyset European woman was sunning herself near my cabana, making a career out of getting the ultimate tan, rotating, wiggling and flipping to get maximum rays. When she arose some hours later, I noticed something very peculiar. She had glaring white crescent moons under her cellulite-ridden butt cheeks. The sun was unable to tan the areas where her bottom had folded over onto itself. I began to wonder if my own backside looked like that.

This story emphasizes a point. We look at everyone else's rear ends but rarely our own. Usually that means "out of sight out of mind." This probably explains why buns look so grim these days as their owners sadly neglect them. So the question is born: "What does a beautifully built backside look like?"

do you think about your butt?

Taking my question to the street, I asked a middle-aged woman what she thought about butts. "Women don't have butts. The boobs go first and then the butt goes. As long as it's flat and not sticking out, it's fine," was her response. "Actually, I don't think about butts that much, but my teenaged daughter certainly does."

Checking out the younger woman's response revealed much more on the subject. Young women are aware that bottoms come in various shapes and that some curves are the result of genetics. If their mothers had generous hips and backsides then the daughters inherited the same. If a flat, skinny butt was a family trait then the daughter would also have a flat, skinny butt. You could end up with a bubble butt or a saggy butt.

Sad to say but most young women felt that butts were on the whole imperfect, but knew enough that a good butt was fat-free. When asked which stars had good bottoms, they readily mentioned **Jennifer Aniston** and **Charlize Theron**.

fast food begets fat butts

The female butt has suffered from neglect with a general demise to this much-misunderstood muscle. When asked what contributed to this downturn, the response, unanimously, was "fast food!" This comes as no surprise. North Americans now eat fast food at a rate that staggers the mind. McDonald's has a marketing goal that targets you, the fast-food eater, to visit the Golden Arches twenty times per month. It's frightening to think that corporate suits actually sit around and discuss how they can manipulate you in such a way as to compel you to eat their greasy food. And the more you eat, the more you gain. That's how North Americans got their super-sized, misshapen butts.

Corporate suits actually sit around and discuss how they can manipulate you to eat their greasy food.

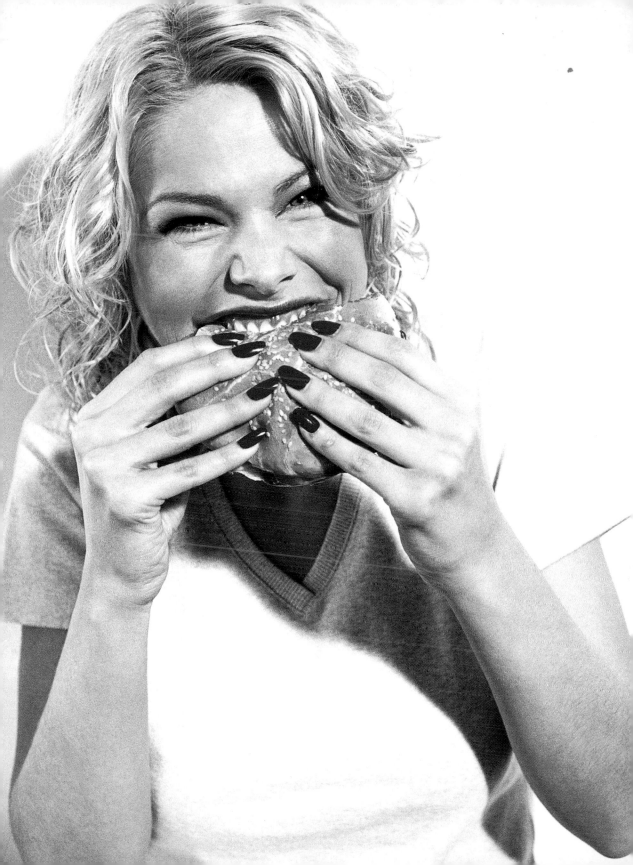

genetics and fruit

In spite of your genetics you can reshape your behind to create what is known in the fitness industry as the apple butt. This kind of behind sits high up on the leg, and is toned, round and free of fat. **Apple butts** are not large. They come in a narrow, tight little package, one that has no trouble sitting in an airplane seat. The apple butt is the ideal shape to strive for.

We recognize that there are other kinds of butt shapes, like the version that belongs to the long-distance runner or the endurance athlete. These buns are highly efficient machines that propel an athlete over long distances. Not an ounce of extra weight here. Then there is the other kind of butt sometimes referred to as the childbearing butt, which is best described as having a tiny waist and large curvaceous hips. There is also a pear-shaped backside, which is a moderately sized set of cheeks that hang low and are not well shaped. Our tanned European gal had this butt package.

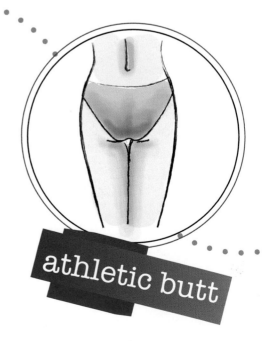

apple butt

athletic butt

This discussion would not be complete without mentioning the mega-sized butt that we are seeing more and more. These back ends are so big that their owners have difficulty buying clothes, or getting in and out of chairs, and don't look even remotely sexy. They look very much like the huge amounts of food that have been poured into creating such gigantic rears – cookies, cakes and pastries. At the other extreme, there is the skinny caboose with no curves at all. These belong to the waifs in the *Sports Illustrated* swimsuit issue or the Victoria's Secret catalogue. The lingerie looks sexy and the swimsuits are hot but the buns are shapeless.

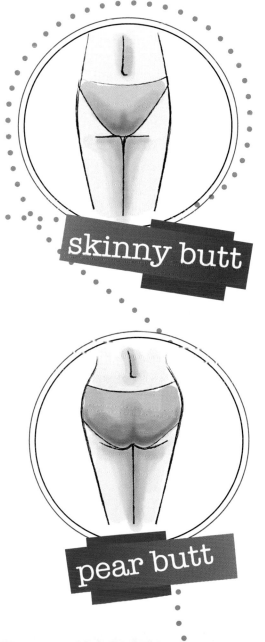

skinny butt

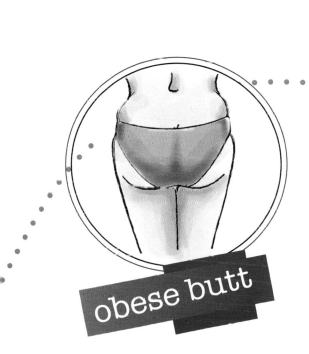

obese butt

pear butt

where can i get a wonder butt bra?

In spite of the ballooning butt and shapeless-rear-end syndrome, women still desire a nice derriere. Many unusual things are tried in order to boost the bottom, most unrelated to diet or physical fitness. Saggy-bunned ladies can now purchase the Biniki, a lace-up bra for their back end. Resembling the jockstrap, thick elastic bands hoist the cheeks up from below. You may also wish to consider the Wonder Butt Bra that accomplishes the same gravity-defying effect as the Biniki. Next time you are flipping through a Victoria's Secret catalogue, check out the butt-boosting undies among the other unmentionables. If any of these options are too binding for you, consider investing in the purchase of a pair of designer pants by Theory. Made with Lycra, Theory pants are all the rage among those in-the-know consumers who simply must own a pair for their magical ability to lift the buttocks and round them out. They are flying off the shelves as women seek to beautify from behind.

get real and get glutes

Snake-oil fixes like these are helpful if a woman doesn't want to tackle the real problem. Glutes need a realistic exercise regimen and proper diet to be at their flattering best. The shape of your bottom is directly affected by your diet and lifestyle. With a careful approach to eating that includes only clean foods, you will accomplish at least ninety percent of your butt-beautifying goal. You can't really expect to keep indulging in ice cream and hope to have a great behind. It's impossible. The truly great backside is born from high-quality foods like lean chicken and fish, egg whites, fresh fruits and vegetables, nutritious grains like rice and oatmeal and loads of pure water. This kind of diet produces a bottom that looks more like the firm red apple you should be eating.

To get it dead right and lifted sky high on your backside where it ought to be, you need to work the glutes too. They're big strong muscles. They can take it. Cardio alone is not enough. Cardio will help if you have only a few pounds to remove. To maximize results, lift weights. Lift weights and lift more weights. Don't worry about getting bulky muscles. You didn't worry about getting a bulky, fat butt, did you? Women don't have enormous amounts of circulating testosterone in their blood so they simply can't get massive. However, they certainly can get toned and tight. Wouldn't it be nice to trade your size 16 Levi's for a pair of size 8s?

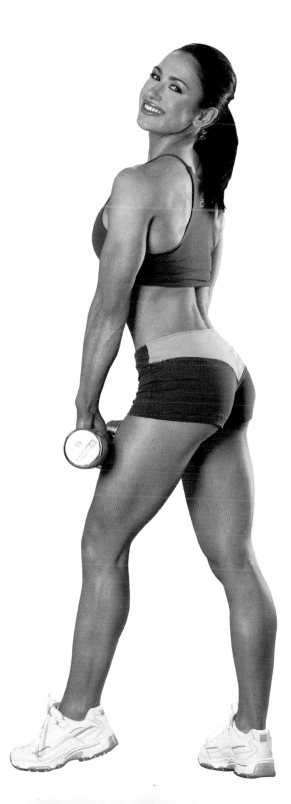

Did You Know?

A list of synonyms for the *buttocks*.

- Arse
- Ass
- Backside
- Behind
- Bum
- Butt
- Buttocks
- Can
- Cheeks
- Derriere
- Fanny
- Glutes
- Gluteus Maximus
- Gluteal Region
- Hiney
- Hind End
- Posterior
- Rear
- Rear End

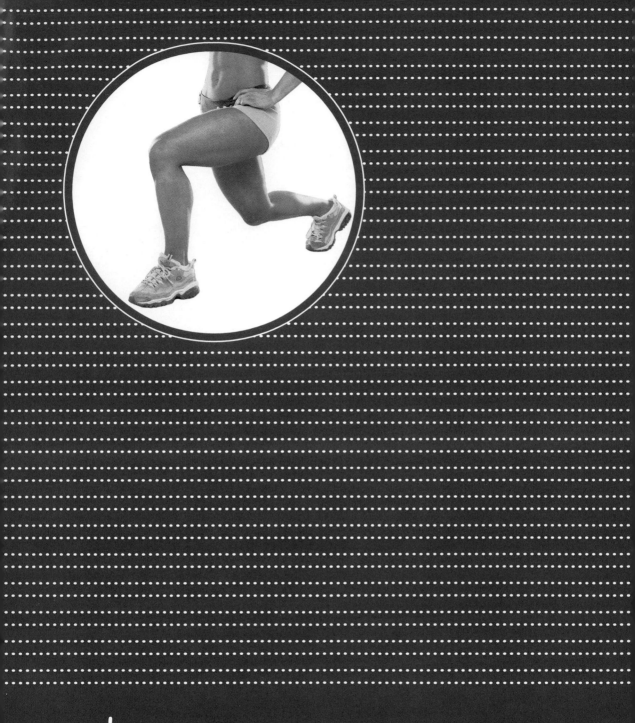

CHAPTER two

five non-apparatus glute exercises + one free mystery exercise

Chances are you are sitting on your duff reading this book right now. That's fine until you get to the end of this piece, but from then on you'll want to kick your can into high gear with these no-fail butt-building moves. No fancy equipment required. No cute little gym outfit or makeup needed. No one to judge the status of your rear while you work it. So grab your water bottle and your energy.

The pursuit of a perfectly polished posterior – tight, round and sky high – is among most women's dreams, ranking at least as important as a pair of beautiful, perky breasts, from an aesthetic point of view. Located on your backside, just out of your view, and acting as a hinge every time you sit, stand or bend over, is the group of muscles called the glutes. Although you may think that the butt is composed mostly of fat, and for some of us this is true, this is not always necessarily so. The fat-to-muscle ratio in your caboose can absolutely be changed so that you are seeing less cottage cheese and much more tightly toned muscle.

Most of your behind is composed of muscle tissue commonly known as the **gluteus maximus**, a wide, thick muscle that wraps around the exterior of the hips and buttocks. It is responsible for extending the leg backward and for rotating the pelvis and thighs. It is one of the body's largest and strongest muscles, capable of lifting hundreds of pounds. The **gluteus medius**, located just above the gluteus maximus, is a smaller muscle that works to raise the leg out and to the side and also helps to keep the body balanced. Dancers have extremely well developed gluteus medius muscles, as they depend upon these for their undeniable grace and skill. The **gluteus minimus** lies under the upper part of the gluteus maximus and works in concert with the gluteus medius. If you want the upper part of your tush to sit higher on your torso, you must focus on the exercises that target the gluteus maximus. If your butt is saggy or droopy you will need to zero in on the minimus and maximus muscles at the same time.

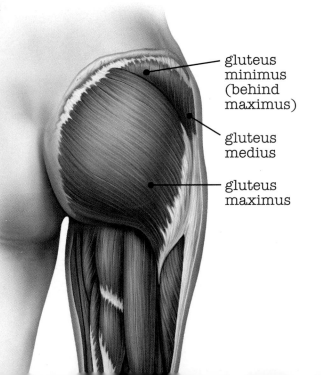

gluteus
minimus
(behind
maximus)

gluteus
medius

gluteus
maximus

Not everyone can get to a gym to start blasting away at butt exercises. Sure, we all make excuses but it is true that gym memberships are expensive and you might not have a way to get around. Then there are those of you who are innately shy about performing glute exercises at all, especially in a gym with many eyes upon you as you sweat your way through your workout. *The Butt Book* comes to your rescue with this athlete-tested list of glute exercises, guaranteed to deliver firm buns. This list of six non-apparatus butt exercises will give you and your cheeks the booty makeover you have been searching for.

Women tend to put weight on in the hips and buttocks area, unlike men who pack it on their middles. Good news though! Women have an upper edge when it comes to training because they have a higher pain tolerance than men and don't grumble as much when it comes to getting the job done.

Glute muscles respond best to consistent training. Several exercises targeting a specific group of muscles must be performed. This way the muscle group, in this case the glutes, is challenged from many different angles, which encourages maximum results. Are you ready for this? Get your backsides in gear because we are gonna get busy!

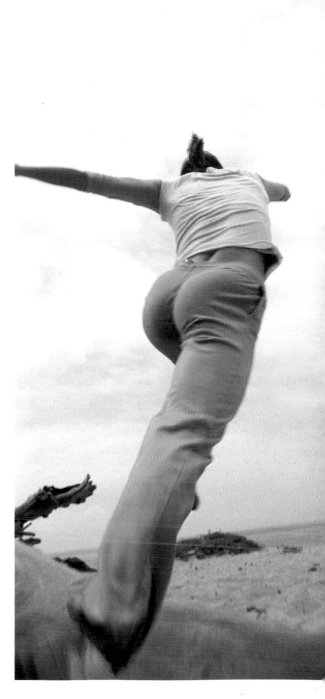

exercise 1
leg raises, or kickbacks

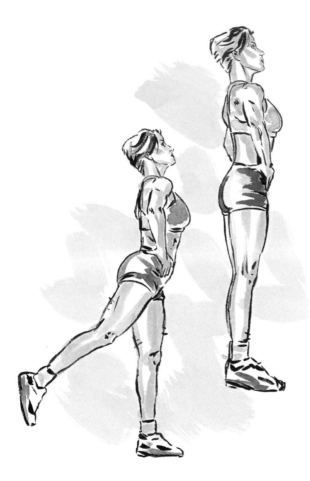

Performing several sets of leg raises or kickbacks without weight will place a demand on the gluteus maximus, especially if they are performed with slow and steady control and with plenty of repetitions – reps for short. Stand feet together, hands on hips. Lift one leg behind you, keeping the torso as upright as possible. For added measure you may occasionally place one hand on the glute as you perform the exercise to feel the muscle working as you raise and lower each leg. Perform fifteen leg raises for each leg. After you have completed one set, take a thirty-second rest and then repeat. If you can, perform a final set. Did you remember to breathe? A well-oxygenated muscle will perform better for you, so keep your breathing strong and deep. Within two to four weeks you should be able to perform three to four sets of these, working up to fifteen reps per set.

❝Don't forget to keep your breathing strong and deep.❞

exercise 2
hip thrusts

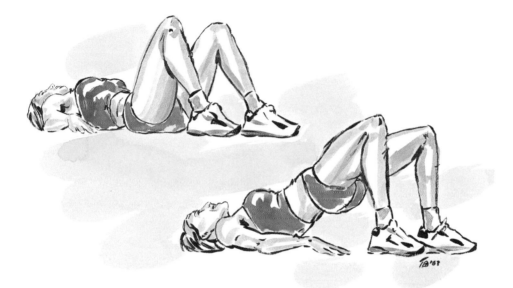

A superb exercise for developing a sky-high bottom, hip thrusts are a must in every woman's butt-building regimen. Fitness athletes perform these with a weight disc on their abdomens for superior results. Find a flat space and lie down on your back on the floor. Place your hands on the floor beside you and draw your knees up, keeping your bottom on the floor. Now raise your bottom up as high as you can, squeezing all the way. In case you are in doubt that the glute muscle is working, place your hand on the upper part of the backside. You should feel a definite tensing of the muscle. Doesn't it feel great? Perform ten reps, squeezing all the way. Do not rest between reps. For a real butt burner try pulsing the movement at the top of the rep. To do this, raise your hips off the floor as high as you can and perform ten small pulses in succession. Alternate these pulses of ten with your full-range hip raises. Work your way up to three to four sets of these, performing 15 to 30 reps. This is an excellent exercise for creating the apple bottom of your dreams.

exercise 3
squats

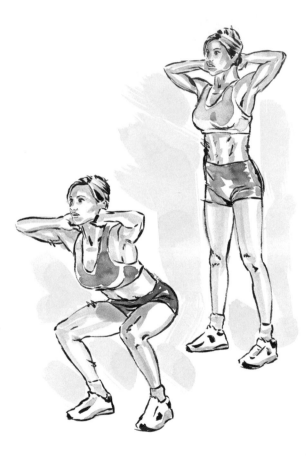

Squats have long been favored as the ultimate butt-building, and incidentally, quad-building exercise. This basic form of squat performed with a flat back in good style is ideal for rounding out the glutes. For women, the squat works the entire leg and glute area without adding bulk. It is not a good idea to skip this one so let's go. Standing with legs shoulder width apart and hands on hips, sink slowly to the ground until your thighs are parallel to the floor. Keep your back flat and your head up. Hold for a count of two, squeezing at all times, and then rise up to the starting position. Repeat for 8 to 10 reps, performing three sets. Never squat too far below parallel, as it is not required for optimal butt-building results. You may also like to try the wide-stance squat for variation. Place your feet way out to the side, as much as two feet apart, toes pointed out. Lower into a full squat position, remembering to breathe deeply in and out each repetition. (Breathe in on the way down, out on the way up.)

As in the case of the regular squat you should keep your back flat throughout the exercise, and lower to the point where your upper legs are parallel to the floor.

> " For women, the squat works the entire leg and glute area without adding bulk. "

exercise 4
walking lunges

Ah lunges! They deliver backside results like few other exercises can. When you get to be a pro at these, you'll be able to perform them holding five-pound weights, and then ten and then twenty. There will be no stopping you. As an added benefit, lunges not only work the entire set of glutes, but will help you develop a more beautifully defined pair of legs too. What are you waiting for? Stand with legs together and hands on hips. Keep knees soft and contract that bottom of yours. Take a step forward with the left leg. Leaving the left foot flat on the floor, bend the back knee – that's on the right leg – toward the floor. But don't touch the floor. Return to the starting position and repeat with the alternate leg. You should be able to perform 8 to 10 repetitions of these for each leg per set, doing three sets with 40-to 60-second breaks in between. If you are feeling more of a burn in the quads, it's because you are making the quads do all the work. What you really want is the glutes to do it. Try placing your hand on your backside to feel the muscle contracting. You will get better results this way.

As an added benefit, lunges not only work the entire set of glutes, but will help you develop a more beautifully defined pair of legs too.

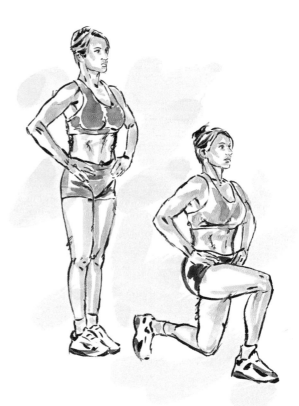

exercise 5
mule kicks on knees

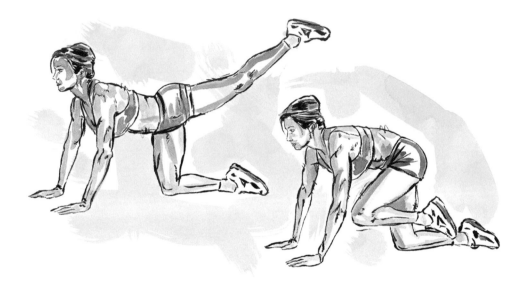

When you get the beautiful rear you want, you will be glad that you added mule kicks to your program. Are you having fun yet? Start by getting on your hands and knees. No, we are not going to wash the floor. Make sure that your back is flat, head is up, elbows are locked and your feet and knees are together. With foot flexed and knee bent, lift your leg as high as you can, squeezing your rear end. Hold it! Hold it! Yes, hold it for a count of two and then draw the leg down and under you to your chest. Repeat this motion for ten counts. Then do it again for the other leg. Complete three sets of these, performing 10 to 15 reps per set. You should really feel that contraction as you raise and lower your legs. This is another excellent way to hit the entire group of glute muscles.

exercise 6
mystery exercise

We are so sure that these exercises will work for you as your create the backside you have always wanted that we are including a freebie. Here's an exercise you can do any time you are walking. Any time! With every stride you take while you are out running errands, walking the dog or doing the groceries, contract the glute muscle. Giving your buns a tight squeeze each time you take a step will add beautiful definition and tone to your other end. This is an exercise that is so easy to do, there's no excuse not to. Best of all no one but you will know you are doing it. So come on ladies, get squeezing and walk your way to a tightly toned tush.

the bottom end

A program of exercises like these along with a clean diet of high-quality foods including grilled chicken, fresh fruits and vegetables and plenty of water will go a long way towards developing your defined derriere. A great ass is not God given. Genetics will only get you so far, but thanks to our tried-and-true tush-training program combined with clean eating, you will be the owner of a backside to be proud of. So put us to the test.

My own dreams for a better backside were realized by following just such a program.

I was amazed that someone like me with basically no butt at all could change my shape completely with just a little extra effort. That is why I know for sure that if you embrace this Butt-Building Program with all the tenacity and power that lies within you, you too will experience results you've only dreamed of.

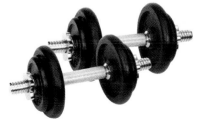

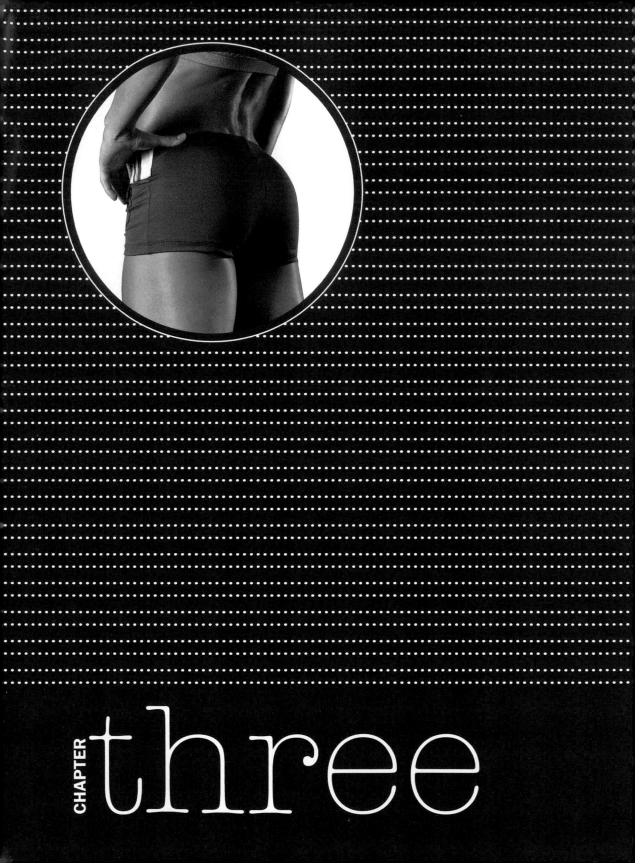

CHAPTER three

building
better
buns

You've noticed that including butt exercises without weights in your training regimen has produced noticeable results. Maybe you've lost several pounds or inches and you're still glowing from the endorphin rush. You feel healthy and alive again. Bolstered by this success and the promise of a truly divine derriere, you begin to toy with the idea that you want more. You've seen some of the fitness women who have amazingly rounded glutes. How do you get those?

Now you're ready to move on to the free-weight section of the gym. Cardio is fine for starting the butt-building process but it can't deliver the built buns you really desire.

Hanging your ego on the door, you plunge ahead regardless of the little twinge of apprehension you might feel working out with the big boys and all of that heavy weight-lifting equipment. Never mind. It's too tempting – you do want the butt of your dreams and you know the only way to get it is with weights. Weights are to your glutes what a pickaxe is to a mountaineer. They're essential for stripping away excess fat and boosting your glute muscles sky high. Exercising with weights carves curves out of fat, shapeless bottoms like no other training regimen ever could.

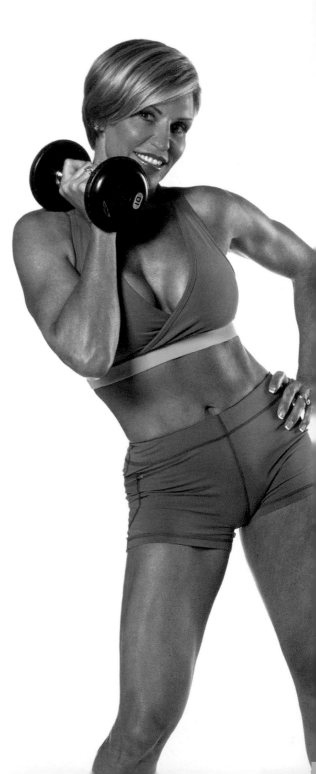

With the image of a shiny, apple-shaped shimmy clearly pictured in your mind, or better yet, posted on your bathroom mirror, throw your arsenal of gym shoes, water bottle, protein shakes and workout gear into your gym bag and get busy building your beautiful booty now!

The following glute exercises, performed with weights and resistance, are the choice of fitness pros and smart readers like you who recognize a good thing when they see it. Proven to deliver the best and most direct butt-shaping results, you will want to include these in your training regimen right away. So let's roll.

squats **are not for gorillas**

You must learn to love squats. Performed correctly, squats will endow you with the best backside results when redesigning your glutes. Many of us have flat, even non-existent backsides that must be coaxed into curviness by performing the regular back squat. As an added bonus, the basic back squat will work the entire leg and glute area and will recharge your metabolism. What are you waiting for?

Since women do not have high amounts of testosterone circulating in their blood,

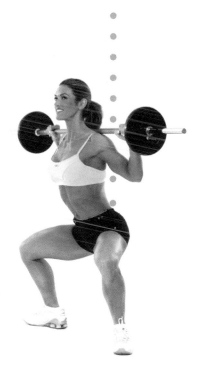

Squats will endow you with the best backside results.

there is no danger of developing huge, out-of-proportion backsides. The basic squat is your friend. Learn it and love it. I promise you won't look like a muscle-bound gorilla.

Place a barbell across your shoulders, choosing a weight that is reasonable for you and your strength level. This is no time to break records, so do not squat with heavy weights just yet. The barbell should be taken from a special "squat rack" to avoid having to lift it and hoist it over your head to place across your shoulders. When performing the squat, keep your back flat, your head up and lower your backside slowly to the floor. Aim for the "thigh just below parallel to the floor" position. Do not bounce out of a squat. All movements are slow, studied and steady. As you rise up out of the squat, squeeze the glutes tightly and stick them out behind you for added butt-building results. By using a wider stance with toes pointed out, all of your effort will be placed on the glutes, challenging them to the maximum.

Perform three sets of squats, doing 12 to 15 reps in each set. Remember to breathe deeply between each repetition – your glute muscles will be screaming for oxygen and deep breathing helps. Between sets do straight-arm pullovers to regain a more normal breathing pattern and to put oxygen back into the muscle. Use a very light weight for these.

As an excellent added benefit, including squats in your butt-training regimen will kickstart your metabolism, rousing it to a higher fat-burning level. What a bonus!

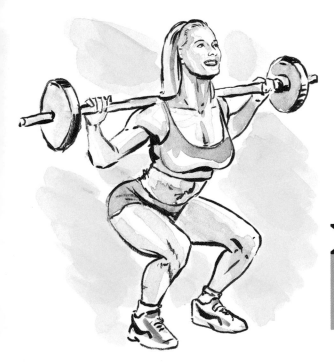

squats

sets: 3
reps: 12-15

walking lunges –
the super performer

The walking lunge, performed with weights, lifts your sloppy backside muscles to new heights. Lunges can be executed with either a barbell weight across the shoulders or with dumbbell weights in both hands. In either case, start with a reasonable weight so that you can perfect your technique first. Don't reach for a 45-pound dumbbell yet. Start with a pair of 5's or 10's.

The lunge requires you to be totally focused on your glute muscles as you perform each repetition since it is primarily a thigh exercise. You'll know what I mean when you start feeling the burn in your thighs instead of in the glutes. Put your mind into the muscle – think butt building. Change the thigh burn to a butt burn by squeezing the glute muscle throughout the entire movement.

A common mistake with the lunge occurs when you overextend the movement so that you are leaning out way over the toe. Knees must never move out past the toes, as this places unnecessary stress on the knee and does nothing to enhance your efforts. Lunge forward until the lower leg forms a slightly sharper than ninety degree angle with the floor. The leg beneath the knee is parallel to the floor. To finish, pull the following leg forward as you begin to rise. Make your way across the gym floor, repeating the lunge until you have completed 20 repetitions – 10 for each leg. Resting between each set, perform four sets of walking lunges.

If you have been concentrating on squeezing those glutes of yours, you will definitely feel your efforts. Lunges work wonders with most behinds so don't neglect to include these in your workout.

walking lunges

sets: 4
reps: 20

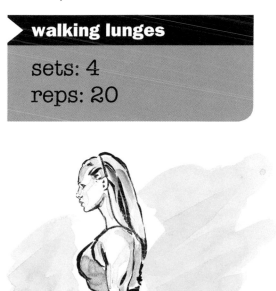

stiff-leg deadlifts **for dummies**

The stiff-leg deadlift is a butt-building exercise loved by all the pros wanting not just deadly buns but exceptional ones. It is the one exercise that works both the glutes and the hamstrings, creating the lovely S-curve on the back of the leg that only elite athletes have. The sinewy curve of the hamstring perfectly balances the outrageous curve of the backside.

The stiff-leg deadlift must be performed with a flat back. When in the lower position the back is particularly vulnerable and open to injury. Keep the back flat and the head up, with the knees slightly bent in order to avoid injury. Standing on a bench, stick your backside out and grip a barbell in front of you. No heavy weights are to be used in this exercise either. The idea is to work the glute muscles with a reasonable weight and to perform more repetitions. With the barbell in your hands, lower your torso so that the weight just reaches the floor but does not touch it. Feel the stretch in your hamstrings and in your glutes. The weight is never thrust forward, rather it moves directly up and down as you raise and lower your torso. Do not rest the weight on the floor between repetitions.

It may be necessary to "spot" by keeping the eyes focused on a spot directly on the floor in front of you so you don't get dizzy. Dancers use this technique when they are performing pirouettes. As you improve, your flexibility also improves, allowing you to lower the barbell below the bench you are standing on.

stiff-leg deadlifts

sets: 3
reps: 10-12

low-cable kickbacks for extreme results

For a highly specialized glute attack, try low-cable kickbacks for extreme results. Often performed in a standing position, even more butt burn can be accomplished in this novel kneeling position.

Place a bench near a low pulley and attach one ankle to the pulley. Select a weight that is reasonable for you. Now is not the time to go for heavy weights. Higher repetitions with lighter weights deliver the best results. Kneeling on the bench with one leg, and the other attached to the pulley, start with the attached leg well forward. Using deliberate control, pull the leg backwards employing the "mind into the muscle" squeeze. Beautiful backsides are not built by staring out the window daydreaming, you must think your way through the movements. Raise the attached leg back behind you as high as possible, feeling the glute involvement as it pumps. Slowly lower back to the beginning position. It is just as important to use slow, deliberate movements on the way down so that the glute is challenged at all times during the back-and-forth movement. Repeat this movement for 12 to 15 reps. As you progress you may perform as many as 25 reps. Complete three sets for each leg.

Low-cable kickbacks hit the glute muscle way up high on the backside helping to lift the butt into a rounder, higher curve.

low-cable kickbacks

sets: 3
reps: 12-15

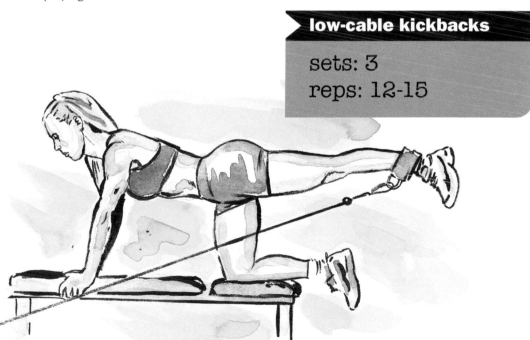

hip thrusts **with weight –** *what?*

For the dedicated among you, be sure to include hip thrusts with weight in your butt-blasting routine, as the ultimate exercise to carve that curve into your backside. Not for the shy or weak at heart, the hip thrust can be a little intimidating since it requires you to place upwards of 35 pounds of weight on your tummy and then lift it skywards. Have I gotten your attention yet?

Lie down on your back on an exercise mat. Have a plate nearby so that you can easily lift it onto your tummy. Don't start with a heavy weight until you perfect your technique and build up your strength. Once you are comfortable, grasp the weight and place it on your tummy. Draw your knees up with feet firmly planted on the floor under your buns. Now raise your hips and squeeze those glute muscles as you lift. Then lower your hips to the ground but do not rest on or touch the ground. Instead, repeat the hip thrust motion ten times. You should feel the glute muscles working hard, high up on your backside. Do three more sets of hip thrusts, increasing the repetitions up to 20 reps per set. In the last set, after you have performed your first 15 to 20 reps, do not rest but keep your hips raised high and perform what is called the "burns." The "burns" are tiny pulses, no more than four to five inches in range, performed at the top of the movement. There is no question that you will feel the burn and what a wonderful feeling that is!

hip thrusts with weight

sets: 3
reps: 15-20

the well-kept butt-building secret

Prone hyperextensions are a well-kept butt-building secret. Experienced pros know the value of this exercise, originally performed to build and strengthen the lower back, for developing a to-die-for derriere.

A specialized machine allows the legs to be stationary while the upper body is free to move up and down. Place your hands behind your head and slowly lower and lift your upper body, focusing on squeezing the glutes all the way. Do not swing back and forth rapidly. Instead use controlled movements to steadily lower the body to the floor and then rise until the body is in a straight line. Lower and repeat for 12 to 15 reps per set and perform three sets. You may need to spot or concentrate on one spot on the floor in front of you, in order to prevent dizziness. In time as the muscles strengthen, you may add a barbell behind your neck or you may use a plate clasped to your chest in front of you.

It's now been a few days since your butt-building bonanza began and you are reminded of it with every step you take. Each step requires the glutes to do their job and while your glutes are working you experience DOMS – delayed onset muscle soreness. But it's a pain to be proud of because you are now among the elite who work their buns like the pros. Pain means progress.

I do not recommend that you do all these butt exercises in one workout. Select just three and perform them twice a week. You can change around your selection every so often so that your butt muscles are constantly challenged with variety. Now where did you put that ideal-butt picture?

prone hyperextensions

sets: 3
reps: 12-15

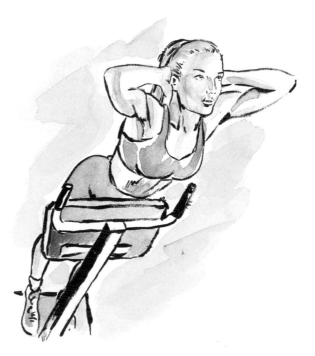

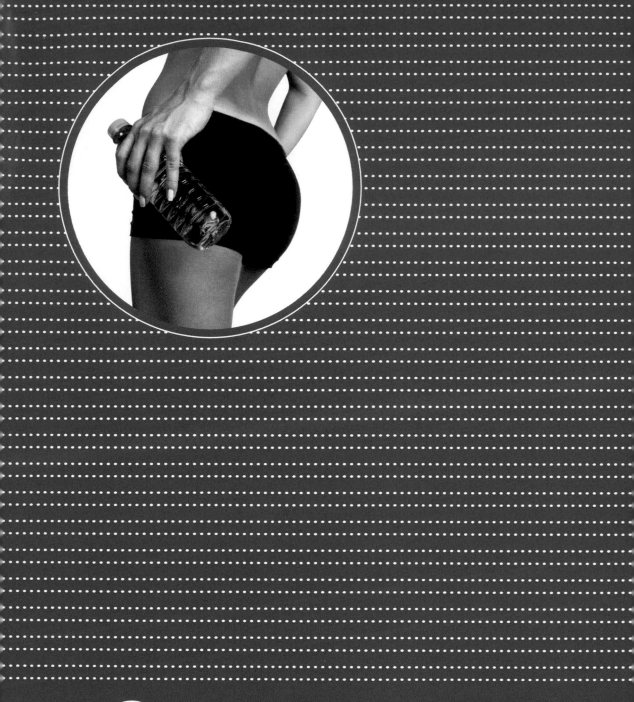

CHAPTER four

the butt that diet built

→ *"I like big butts and I cannot lie."*

→ Sample One-Day Eating Plan

→ Your Eating Discipline

❝Realize this—great butts don't come just from training. Nutrition counts, too.❞

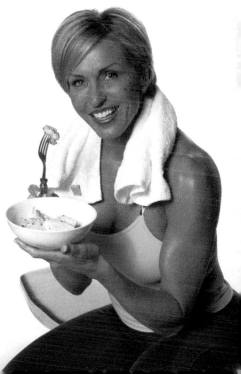

"I like big butts and I cannot lie."

—lyrics from Sir Mix-a-Lot

This popular tune picks up on the notoriety buttocks have been receiving lately. Jennifer Lopez has a posterior that is the envy of many and Madonna's rear end was paid a handsome sum for advertising GAP jeans with Missy Elliot. With all the limelight focused on the behind, a girl has to be prepared by getting her own particular curves to be at her bodacious best.

Most of us dream of possessing a great ass but we are not always born with one. Over and above simple genetics a sexy, round, toned butt must be created through a combination of diet and exercise. What to do? The butt is often overlooked when it comes to training but it is the strongest muscle group in the body, enabling you to lift hundreds of pounds. Contrary to popular belief, exercise and weight training alone are not the quick fixes for every problem spot on the body. You could exercise and train for years, achieving minimal results. Since bodybuilding, or more accurately, body shaping, is roughly 80 percent nutrition, a controlled diet is impossible to ignore when trying to develop a tightly toned bottom.

Most of us overestimate how controlled our eating program is, so it is important to assess your current eating habits honestly. To achieve the kind of "apple butt" posterior you desire, you need to be as dedicated to your diet as you are to your exercise and weight-training regimen. Every one of us gets the urge to grab a pseudo-nutritious bar of some sort after a truly killer workout in the gym. Already you have sabotaged your own efforts to get good results by indulging yourself in an impulse. The point is, with respect to your food regimen, garbage in equals garbage out.

Let's talk about nutrition – serious, butt-tightening, fat-destroying nutrition. The

• The best high-quality protein sources include only the leanest, cleanest forms of poultry and fish.

body requires high-quality, low-fat, low-sugar nutrients in order to run efficiently. These can be simply grouped into four categories including protein, carbohydrates, fat and water.

Protein is the basic structural tissue of the human body. This primary macronutrient cannot be stored in the body and must be replenished regularly through diet. Lean, strong, sculptural muscles bursting with robust health are built from protein. It is essential to supply the muscles with lean protein sources of energy every two to three hours if you are intent on creating a beautiful backside. The best high-quality protein sources include only the leanest, cleanest forms of poultry and fish. Generally, boneless, skinless chicken breasts, grilled or baked, along with varieties of white fish will form the backbone of this controlled diet. Each time protein is consumed,

some complex carbohydrates should also be consumed, as they facilitate the assimilation of protein in the body. A good protein source for breakfast would be egg whites, either in the form of an omelet or a boiled egg minus the yolk. Other sources of protein to have in moderation include whole unroasted unsalted nuts and protein supplements, including protein drinks or bars. A warning about bars – they can derail your butt-creating efforts if you rely on them too heavily. It's best to establish

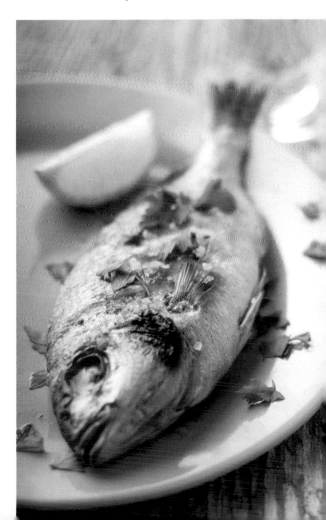

a routine of eating high-quality protein sources like chicken and fish early on. Active people need more protein in their diet, so get busy and eat up. The best-tasting bar, which also delivers 25 grams of protein, is the Meso-Tech bar, but for added butt muscle you can't beat the Nitro-Tech bar. It contains a full 35 grams of protein and when combined with the butt-building diet and weight-training program, is the protein bar supreme.

But protein is useless if you don't eat carbohydrates too. Yes, carbohydrates must

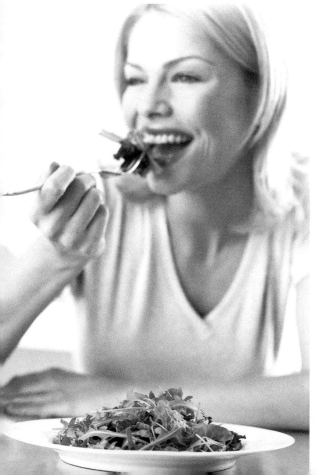

be consumed as they facilitate the body's protein absorption. Remember, muscle consists of protein. You want to consume protein and build muscle efficiently in order to develop the backside of your dreams. Consuming certain types of carbohydrates will pay off in your pursuit. There are two kinds of carbohydrates, simple and complex. Simple carbohydrates contain little to no fiber and encourage an insulin surge or sugar rush after they have been consumed. Simple carbohydrates are normally found in refined sugars and fruit juices. Carbohydrates like these are among the first foods you must remove from your diet and avoid at all costs. You won't get an apple butt by devouring a box of Krispy Kremes chased by a Coke. Instead choose complex carbohydrates, which are more slowly absorbed by the body and are the primary macronutrient source of energy. Without inducing an insulin surge, complex carbohydrates such as a salad, carrot or whole grains are burned as glucose, which is always present in the blood, and are stored in the liver as glycogen. Fruits and vegetables are the best source of complex carbohydrates as they produce energy for longer periods of time. It is important to know that all sugars count as simple carbohydrates and too many of them will be stored as fat. For women fat is usually stored on the hips and backside. Not ideal if you're trying to build a round, firm bottom.

The primary macronutrient that is the source for long-term energy and energy storage is fat. Some fat is essential to the body, as it facilitates the transport and absorption of fat-soluble vitamins. Also, the human brain consists of highly specialized cells whose function depends on specific fats. The jiggly sags on your lower buttocks and thighs are one hundred percent excess fat, stored away by the body in case of future starvation situations. Given that this is unlikely to occur any time soon and that you want to lift and tone that rear, fat consumption must be addressed with some care. Biochemically there are two kinds of fat – *saturated* and *unsaturated*. *Saturated fats* are solid at room temperature. Think of a pound of butter. These fats are linked to heart disease, stroke and obesity. Keep the consumption of saturated fats to an absolute minimum. *Unsaturated fats* are derived mainly from plant sources and are in a liquid state at room temperature. Keep the consumption of these fats to a minimum as well, although of the two, these are healthier.

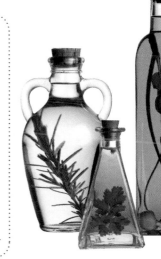

▶unsaturated fat

No discussion on a clean, controlled diet would be complete without discussing water, since it forms a major part of every tissue in the body, including gluteal muscle. We all need to consume plenty of water, more so if we are active and on a butt-building mission. Water is the medium in which most bodily functions are performed, and it is involved in all metabolic reactions. Water carries vital materials to and away from cells.

In order to change the shape of your glutes, you must adopt a controlled eating regimen and include resistance training along with some cardiovascular exercise in your butt-beautifying strategy. In so doing you will eliminate unwanted body fat and uncover the tightly toned tush of your dreams. Paying attention to all of these principles will guarantee results by perfecting not only your posterior but the rest of you too.

◀saturated fat

your
eating guidelines

START YOUR DAY

* Start your day with **large-flake long-cooking oatmeal** (*not instant*)

* Add **berries** for antioxidant power

* Eat an **egg-white omelet** prepared with 4 or 5 egg whites

* Add lightly cooked **vegetables** for flavor if desired

* Use a non-stick pan or PAM **cooking spray**

* Drink **clear green tea** or **black coffee** without sweetener

* Supplement with **vitamins,** especially essential fatty acids and vitamin C

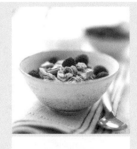
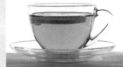
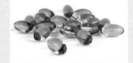

EVERY 2-3 HOURS THROUGHOUT THE DAY

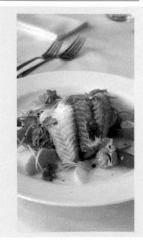

* Eat a **palm-sized** serving of protein – *about 4 or 5 ounces*

* Protein should consist of **clean**, **white** meat as follows – chicken, tuna, turkey, white fish such as sole, snapper or halibut, salmon, and egg whites

* Proteins should be **baked**, **broiled**, **grilled** or **steamed**

* Consume a serving of raw, roasted, grilled or steamed **vegetables** with each protein meal

DINNER

* Dinner follows the same guidelines as meals consumed every two to three hours, but you may add a **small serving of carbohydrates**

* Carbohydrates include **whole-wheat wraps, sweet potatoes, rice and potatoes**

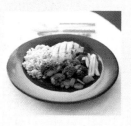

SNACKS

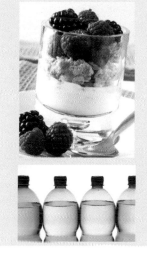

If you must snack, try any of the following in moderation.

* Small handful of unsalted cashews or almonds

* Apples

* Low-fat, plain yogurt mixed with fresh berries or unsweetened applesauce

* Clear, green tea or black coffee

* $\frac{1}{3}$ cup of hot oatmeal

* Water and lots of it

"Healthy snacking may actually prevent you from overeating."

your eating discipline

1 Get used to preparing more food each time you cook. This way you have extra food ready when you need it and you'll need it more often on this clean-eating regimen.

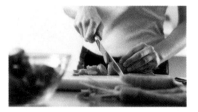

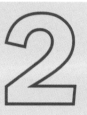

In order to lose weight you will have to eat more good food, *more often*. **2**

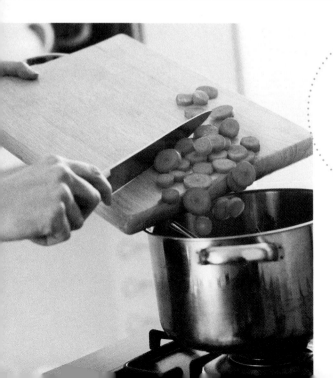

3 Although it takes a little more time to prepare food than to eat food that you bought prepared, it does not mean you have to double your time in the kitchen. Try cooking an extra casserole or more chicken breasts or a large pot of soup. **Keep extra servings in the freezer**. The extras will serve you well.

4

Remember that if you carry your food with you (as you will have to in order to eat five or six times per day) you will not be tempted to eat junk or food that contains too many empty calories.

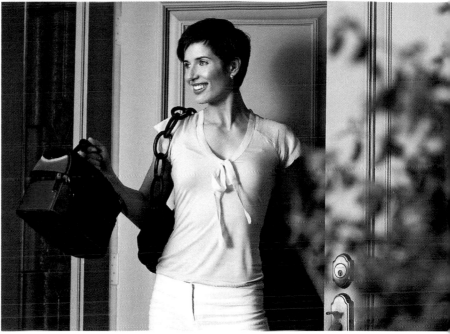

5

Skipping any meal is death to your efforts to achieve a better body.

Get rid of the notion that you should skip breakfast. There are too many studies proving the essential nutritional worth of this critical meal. You have already spent the whole night without food. Your body needs nutrition to kick-start the day properly. What you put in your mouth at breakfast dictates how your day will go and how you'll feel throughout.

6

For more detailed information on eating clean, pick up a copy of my book **The Eat-Clean Diet**. Go to www.toscareno.com or www.eatcleandiet.com.

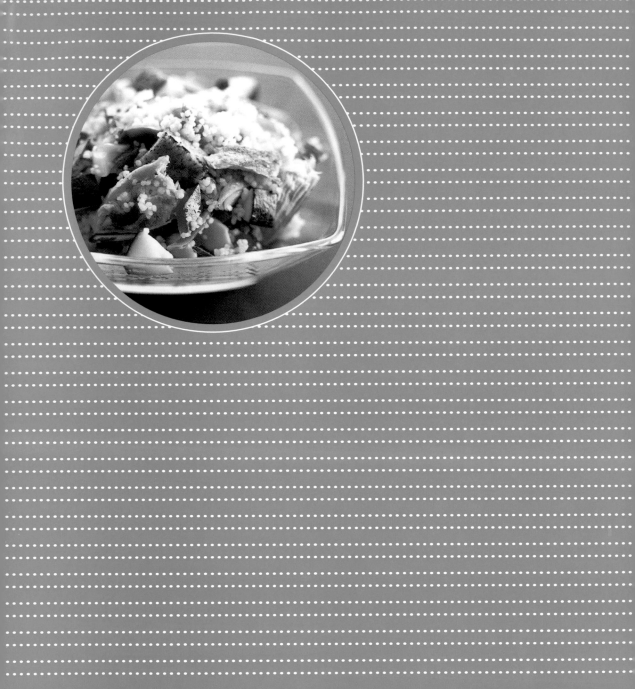

one week of clean-eating menus

DAY ONE

Meal #1

BREAKFAST – 7:00 am

→ ⅔ cup cooked oatmeal topped with ¼ cup blueberries or raspberries

→ 3 or 4 hardboiled eggs without the yolks

→ 1 piece of dry brown toast

→ Black coffee or clear green tea

→ 2 cups water

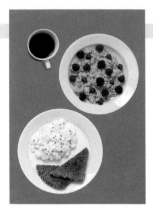

Meal #2

10:30 am

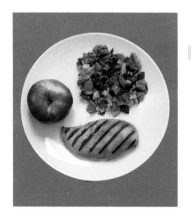

→ 5 ounces of grilled, baked or broiled chicken breast without skin or fat

→ 1½ cup chopped green salad with tomatoes, cucumbers, carrots and radishes

→ 1 apple

→ 1 cup water

Meal #3

1:00 pm

→ 1 or 2 cups **Tomato and Roasted Garlic Soup**
See recipe on page 93

→ Whole-grain wrap

→ 1 whole orange

→ 1 cup water

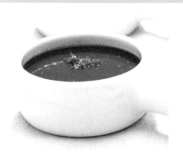

Meal #4

3:30 pm

→ Tuna salad with lemon juice in whole-wheat wrap

→ Carrot sticks, celery sticks, cucumber slices, radishes

→ 2 - 3 wedges of cantaloupe

→ 1 cup water

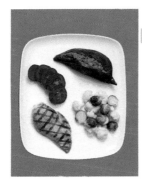

Meal #5

6:00 pm

→ 5 ounce grilled, broiled or baked chicken breast

→ 1 sweet potato, baked – no oil, butter or sour cream!

→ ½ cup each steamed Brussels sprouts and cauliflower

→ Small ripe tomato, sliced, on the side for extra antioxidant power

→ 1 cup water

Meal #6

8:30 pm – This is the last meal of the day!

→ ½ cup cooked oatmeal topped with chopped, peeled apple

→ 1 cup water

→ 1 cup clear green tea

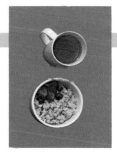

snacks

If you absolutely must have snacks during the day, munch on a handful of unsalted cashews or almonds. Any of these contains protein, which helps to build muscle and both will satisfy your nibbling urges. Don't worry about their high fat content. Nuts contain mostly unsaturated fats, which are beneficial in lowering blood cholesterol levels.

DAY TWO

Meal #1

Breakfast – 7:00 am

→ Egg-white omelet prepared with 5 or 6 egg whites, tomato and spinach
  Hint: *Use Pam or other cooking spray to coat your fry pan.*

→ 1 piece of dry brown toast *(that means no butter or jam)*

→ 1 banana

→ Black coffee or clear green tea

→ 2 cups water

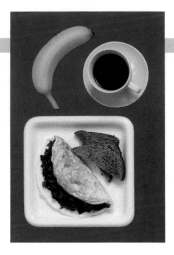

Meal #2

10:30 am

→ Mesclun salad greens with 1 whole apple, thinly sliced

→ ½ cups low-fat cottage cheese

→ 1 cups water

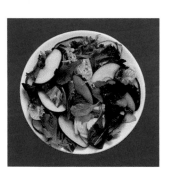

Meal #3

1:00 pm

→ 1 or 2 cups **Spa Vegetable Soup**
  See recipe on page 94

→ 1 whole-grain wrap

→ Sliced cucumbers, sliced red, green and yellow peppers

→ Handful green grapes

→ 1 cup water

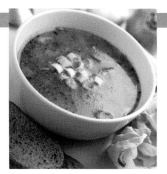

Meal #4

3:30 pm

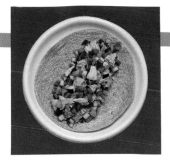

→ Tuna salad with chopped raw veggies and lemon juice

→ 1 whole-grain wrap

→ 2 or 3 slices cantaloupe

→ 1 cup water

Meal #5

6:00 pm

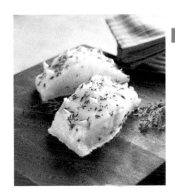

→ **Garlic Herbed Fish**
   See recipe on page 88

→ ½ cup steamed asparagus

→ ½ cup brown rice

→ ½ cup green grapes

→ 1 cup water

Meal #6

8:30 pm

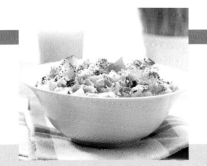

→ **Swiss Muesli**
   See recipe on page 67

→ 1 cup clear green tea

→ 1 cup water

did you notice?

On both **Day One** and **Day Two**, you have been encouraged to drink water with every meal. Drinking enough water is essential to good health and facilitates digestion. *Aren't you feeling better already?*

DAY THREE

Meal #1

Breakfast 7:00 am

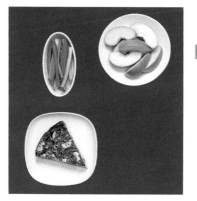

→ ⅔ cup cooked cereal such as buckwheat, quinoa, millet, cream of wheat or oatmeal topped with ¼ cup slivered almonds and ¼ cup dried fruit
Optional: 1 to 2 tablespoons ground flaxseed on oatmeal.

→ 4 hard-boiled egg whites

→ Black coffee or clear green tea

→ 2 cups water

Meal #2

10:30 am

→ **Vegetable Frittata** made with egg whites
See recipe on page 71

→ Carrot and celery sticks

→ 1 whole apple

→ 1 cup water

Meal #3

1:00 pm

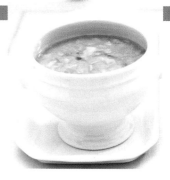

→ 1 or 2 cups of **Leek, Potato and Herb Soup**
See recipe on page 101

→ 1 slice dry whole-grain toast

→ 1 cup water

Meal #4

3:30 pm

→ 5 oz. grilled chicken breast

→ ½ cup steamed green beans

→ ½ yam

→ 1 medium-sized apple

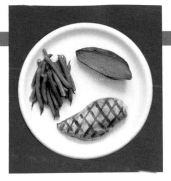

Meal #5

6:00 pm

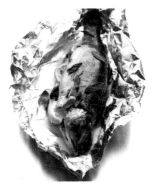

→ **Baked Salmon with Herbs**
   See recipe on page 75

→ ½ cup brown rice

→ 7 or 8 spears steamed asparagus

→ ½ cup steamed carrots

→ 1 cup water

Meal #6

8:30 pm

→ ½ cup cooked oatmeal topped with
   applesauce

→ 1 cup clear green tea

→ 1 cup water

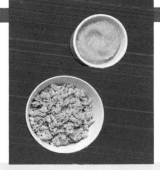

hint

It is worth noting that you are eating more than normal. This is one of the governing principles of clean eating. Eating small meals of high-quality foods more frequently will guarantee the weight-loss results you desire. In other words, you don't have to go hungry!

DAY FOUR

Meal #1

Breakfast 7:00 am

→ 4-egg-white omelet

→ 1 piece dry brown toast

→ 3 watermelon wedges

→ Black coffee or clear green tea

→ 2 cups water

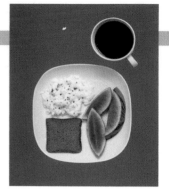

Meal #2

10:30 am

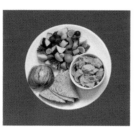

→ Tuna salad on a whole-grain wrap with lemon juice

→ ½ cup raw vegetables

→ 1 whole apple

→ 1 cup water

Meal #3

1:00 pm

→ 1 or 2 cups **White Bean and Collard Green Soup**
See recipe on page 98

→ 1 whole-grain pita wrap

→ 1 cup water

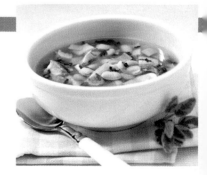

Meal #4

3:30 pm

→ 5 ounces grilled or baked chicken with sliced tomato

→ ½ cup brown rice

→ 2 watermelon wedges

→ 1 cup water

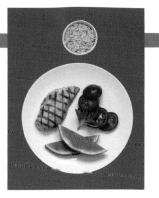

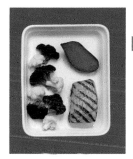

Meal #5

6:00 pm

→ 5 ounces grilled salmon

→ ½ cup steamed cauliflower and broccoli

→ ½ baked yam

→ 1 cup water

Meal #6

8:30 pm

· ½ cup unsalted nuts

· 1 cup clear green tea

· 1 cup water

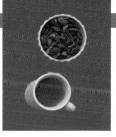

hint

Eating well requires planning and discipline. You may want to prepare extras of certain foods in order to have them ready to eat when you need them. For example, grill several chicken breasts instead of one. This way you will always have some ready for the next meal. Chop enough vegetables for three meals at the same time. Most vegetables keep well for at least two or three days in the refrigerator. Being organized ensures clean-eating success and helps you resist the wrong foods.

DAY FIVE

Meal #1
Breakfast 7:00 am

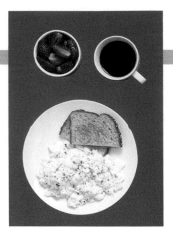

→ ⅔ cup hot oat-bran cereal topped with ½ sliced banana and ½ cup strawberries

→ Egg-white omelet prepared with 5 or 6 egg whites and chopped tomato

→ Black coffee or clear, green tea

→ 2 cups water

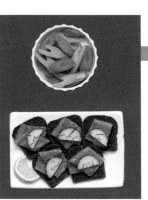

Meal #2
10:30 am

→ 5 or 6 slices smoked salmon with lemon juice

→ 2 slices heavy pumpernickel bread

→ ½ cup celery and carrot sticks

→ 1 cup water

Meal #3
1:00 pm

→ 1 or 2 cups **Curried Pumpkin Soup**
See recipe on page 97

→ 1 whole-grain pita or bagel

→ Assorted crudités: red peppers, cucumbers, carrots, and radish

→ 1 banana or 1 kiwi fruit

→ 1 cup water

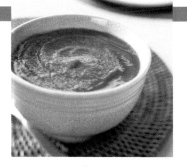

Meal #4
3:30 pm

→ 1 banana with 2 Tbsp nut butter

→ ½ cup unsalted almonds

→ 1 cup water

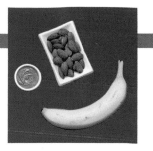

Meal #5
6:00 pm

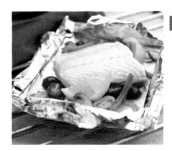

→ **Foil-steamed Spring Vegetables**
See recipe on page 77

→ **Fillet of Sole with Lemon and Parsley**
See recipe on page 77

→ **Smashed Red Potatoes**
See recipe on page 76

→ **Baked Apple**
See recipe on page 67

→ 1 cup water

Meal #6
8:30 pm

→ ½ cup plain low-fat yogurt

→ 1 handful unsalted, unroasted cashews

→ 1 cup clear green tea

→ 1 cup water

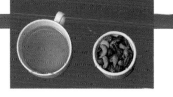

are you still with the program?

Yes it is hard to give up chips and other junk foods if they have been a big part of your previous life. But we don't call it clean eating for nothing. Your pipes are probably plugged up with trans fats, grease and other harmful non-foods that contribute to poor health and obesity. Clean eating works from the inside out, making significant changes that you can't see until the first few pounds disappear. Don't give up just because you can't see the change immediately. You'll feel it before you see it. Stay with us. You can do it!

DAY SIX

Meal #1

Breakfast 7:00 am

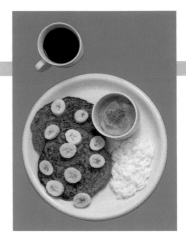

→ 2 **Oatmeal Pancakes** topped with unsweetened apple sauce
See pancake recipe on page 68

→ 1 banana, sliced

→ 2 egg whites, scrambled

→ Black coffee clear green tea

→ 2 cups water

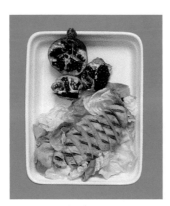

Meal #2

10:30 am

→ 1 pomegranate

→ ½ cup mixed salad greens

→ 5 oz. chicken breast

→ 1 cup water

Meal #3

1:00 pm

→ 1 or 2 cups **Squash Soup Health Purée**
See recipe on page 102

→ 1 whole-grain bagel, toasted

→ 1 whole apple

→ 1 cup water

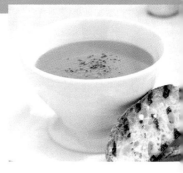

Meal #4

3:30 pm

→ ½ mixed raw vegetables

→ 1 whole-grain wrap

→ 2 oz. low-fat cheese

→ 1 cup water

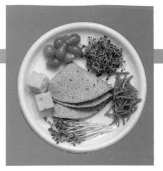

Meal #5

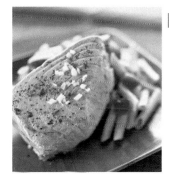

6:00 pm

→ **Seared Tuna**
See recipe on page 79

→ **Roasted Sweet Potato Wedges**
See recipe on page 72

→ ½ cup **Sautéed Baby Bok Choy**
See recipe on page 75

→ ½ cup **Stir-Fried Asparagus, Spinach and Red onion**
See recipe on page 79

→ 1 cup water

Meal #6

8:30 pm

→ ½ cup Muesli

→ 1 cup clear green tea

→ 1 cup water

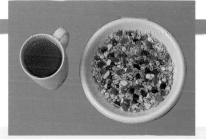

did you forget?

Sometimes you just can't get organized enough to prepare healthy food in advance. Relax. There's help. You can supplement with protein bars like Nitro-Tech and Meso-Tech or protein drinks like Nitro-Tech. These are meant to be used in a pinch, not for every meal.

DAY SEVEN

Meal #1

Breakfast 7:00 am

→ 1 cup oat-bran cereal, cooked

→ ½ cup mixed berries

→ 6-egg-white omelet

→ Black coffee or clear green tea

→ 2 cups water

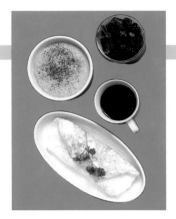

Meal #2

10:30 am

→ 1 apple

→ ½ cup unsalted almonds

→ 2 cups water

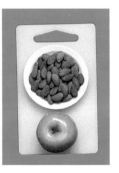

Meal #3

1:00 pm

→ 1 or 2 cups **Bean, Potato and Red Pepper Soup**
See recipe on page 105

→ 1 piece dry whole-grain toast

→ 1 orange

→ 1 cup water

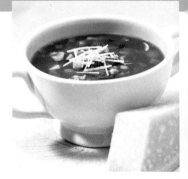

Meal #4

3:30 pm

→ Stir-fried vegetables with chopped, grilled chicken breast

→ Serve in whole-grain wrap

→ 1 apple

→ 1 cup water

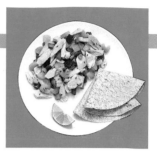

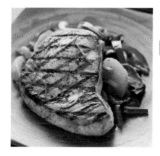

Meal #5

6:00 pm

→ **Lemon-Broiled Swordfish**
See recipe on page 72

→ ½ cup brown rice

→ ½ cup steamed mixed vegetables

→ 1 grapefruit

→ 1 cup water

Meal #6

8:30 pm

→ ½ cup low-fat plain yogurt with mixed berries

→ 1 cup clear green tea

→ 1 cup water

natural gas

Was that you or did the dog do it? Yes you have probably noticed a little more gas than usual. Digesting protein is hard work for the body. Unless you consume the magic combination of protein plus carbohydrates with each meal, you will find that you are more gassy than usual. That is also the reason that it is important to drink at least eight cups of water each day. Don't worry, it will get better as the body gets used to this new way of eating. Until then, just blame it on the dog.

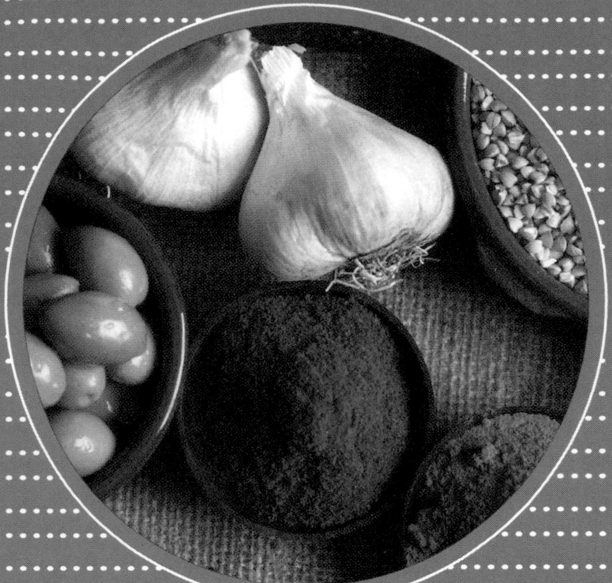

CHAPTER six

one week of clean-eating recipes

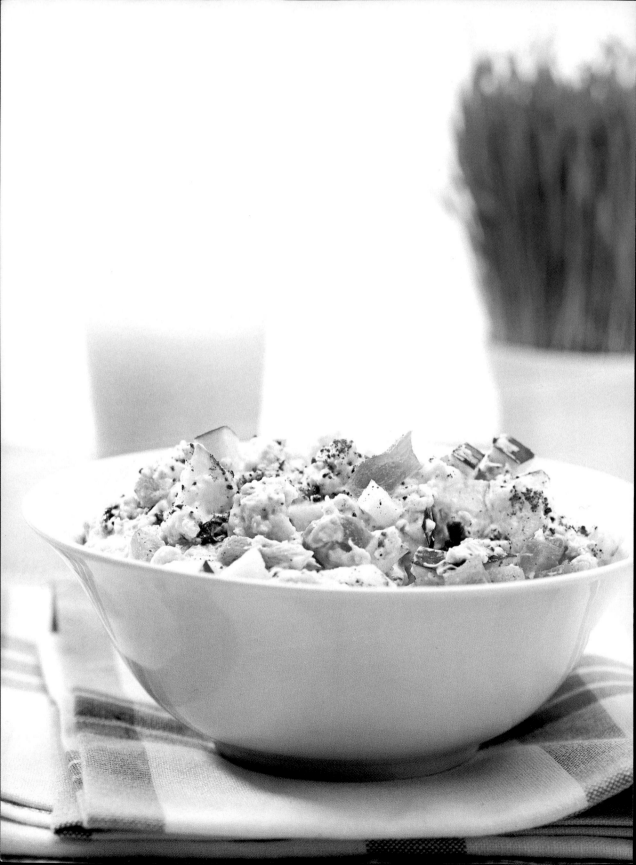

swiss muesli

½ cup	old-fashioned rolled oats, uncooked
½ cup	hot water
1 cup	low-fat or nonfat plain yogurt
¼ cup	raisins, dried cranberries, dried chopped apricots or dried prunes
¼ cup	slivered almonds
2 Tbsp	natural bran
2 Tbsp	oat bran

1. Place oats in small bowl. Pour hot water over oats and let stand for 25 minutes or until all water is absorbed.

2. Add yogurt, dried fruit, almonds, natural bran and oat bran. Mix well. Cover and refrigerate. Keeps for about three days.

3. Add chopped fresh apple, banana or berries for a nourishing breakfast.

Makes 4 servings.

PER SERVING
Calories 257
Protein 7 grams
Fat 2 grams
Carbohydrates 56 grams

baked apple

4	firm apples such as Ida Red, Mutsu or Northern Spy
¼ cup	firmly packed brown sugar
¼ cup	raisins
2 tsp	cinnamon
½ tsp	nutmeg

cooking spray

1 Wash and core apples. Make a shallow cut around the middle of the apple. This will help to prevent the skin from bursting. Place apples in a baking dish that has been lightly coated with cooking spray.

2 In a small bowl, combine remaining ingredients. Put enough water in the baking dish to cover the bottom. Bake apples uncovered in a 375°F oven for about 30 minutes. If apples are very firm you may need to bake them for another 10 to 15 minutes. Apples are tender when pierced with a toothpick. Serve topped with nonfat yogurt.

Makes 4 servings.

PER SERVING
Calories 212
Protein 3 grams
Fat 0.5 grams
Carbohydrates 61 grams

oatmeal pancakes

2½ cups	rolled oats
6	egg whites
1 cup	skim milk soured with one teaspoon lemon juice
1 Tbsp	corn or safflower oil
1 tsp	baking powder
1 tsp	vanilla
cooking spray	

PER SERVING
Calories 600
Protein 28 grams
Fat 16 grams
Carbohydrates 86 grams

1. Place all ingredients in a food processor or a blender and blend for about 20 seconds until smooth.

2. Coat a griddle or a frying pan with cooking spray. Heat pan or griddle until quite hot.

3. Pour ¼ cup pancake batter for each pancake. Cook until pancake edges are dry and bubbles appear on top. Turn and brown the other side. Serve topped with applesauce or sugar-free syrup.

Makes 12 pancakes.

scrambled egg whites

6	egg whites
2 Tbsp	skim milk
¼ tsp	herb seasoning
cooking spray	

PER SERVING
Calories 107
Protein 17 grams
Fat 0.1 grams
Carbohydrates 9 grams

1 In a small bowl combine egg whites, skim milk and seasoning. Whisk until well mixed. Coat a medium frying pan with cooking spray. Heat over medium heat. Pour in the egg mixture.

2 Cook until the egg mixture begins to set at the edges. Using a spatula, stir eggs slowly until they are cooked but still soft. Remove from heat. Serve.

Makes 2 servings.

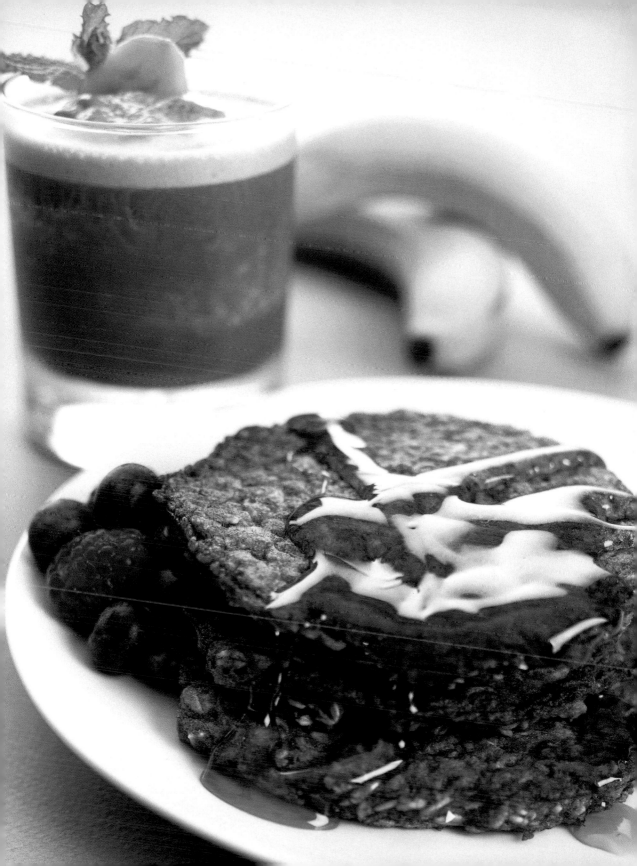

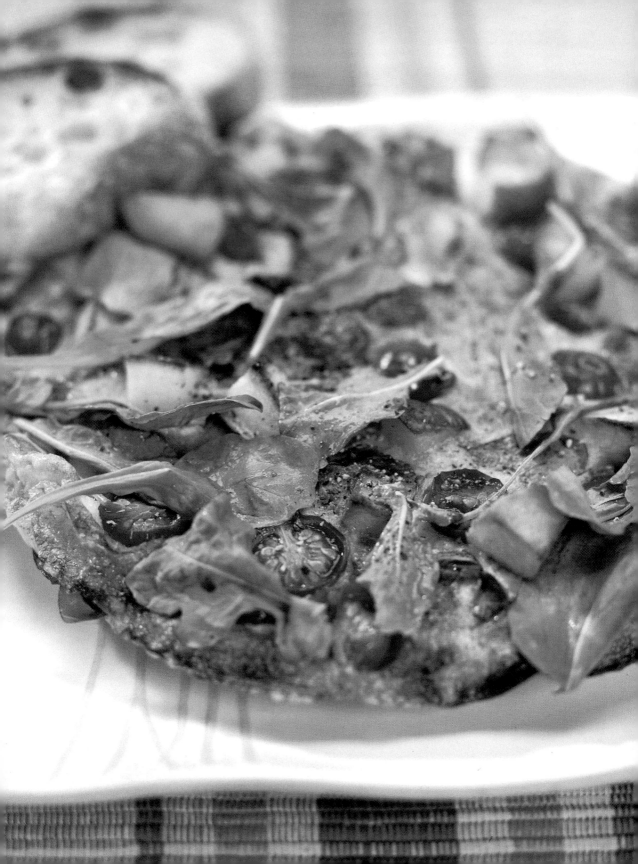

vegetable frittata

1 lb	baby new potatoes
1 Tbsp	olive oil
1	garlic clove, crushed
2 oz	wild rocket (arugula)
6 oz	cloves garlic, minced
8-12	egg whites, beaten

salt and freshly ground black pepper to taste

1. Cut potatoes in half, or into chunks if necessary, then cook in a pot of lightly salted boiling water for 8 to 10 minutes. Drain.

2. Heat oil in a non-stick frying pan. Cook the garlic over low heat for one minute. Scatter the potatoes, half the rocket and the cherry tomatoes into the pan.

3. Pour the eggs on top, season well with salt and freshly ground black pepper and cook over a medium heat for about 5 minutes, until almost set. Use a wooden spatula to lift the frittata so any unset egg can travel to the base of the hot pan.

4. When just set on the bottom, place under a hot broiler grill for 2-3 minutes to set the top. Scatter the remaining rocket overtop and serve.

Makes 4 servings.

PER SERVING
Calories 180
Protein 13 grams
Fat 4 grams
Carbohydrates 23 grams

lemon-broiled swordfish

1 pound	swordfish steaks (about 3 or 4)
2 Tbsp	lemon juice
2 Tbsp	water or dry white wine or combination of both
1 Tbsp	reduced salt soy sauce
2	cloves garlic, minced
¼ tsp	each dried parsley, basil, dill and marjoram
¼ tsp	black pepper

cooking spray

1. Place swordfish in baking dish coated with low-fat cooking spray.

2. Combine all remaining ingredients, except swordfish, in small bowl.

3. Pour marinade over swordfish and allow to marinate for 30 to 40 minutes.

4. Broil fish for five minutes each side, or until fish flakes easily. Use any remaining marinade to baste the fish while broiling.

Makes 4 servings.

PER SERVING
Calories 137
Protein 22 grams
Fat 5 grams
Carbohydrates 0.1 grams

roasted sweet potato wedges

3	sweet potatoes
cooking spray	
½ tsp	chili powder
¼ tsp	salt
¼ tsp	cayenne pepper

1 Preheat oven to 400°F.

2 Scrub sweet potatoes well, trimming off any loose fibers. Cut into 1-inch wedges. Place sweet potatoes in a single layer on a baking sheet sprayed with cooking spray. Lightly mist potato wedges with cooking spray. Sprinkle seasonings over potatoes. Roast in oven for about 35 minutes, stirring occasionally. Sweet potatoes bake more quickly than regular potatoes, so make sure to check them often.

Makes 4 servings.

PER SERVING
Calories 227
Protein 3 grams
Fat 3 grams
Carbohydrates 48 grams

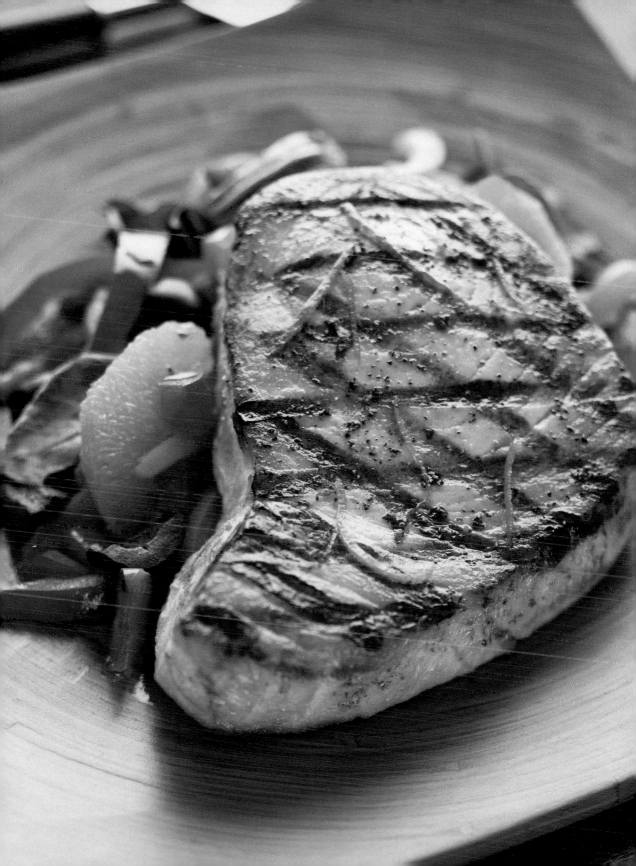

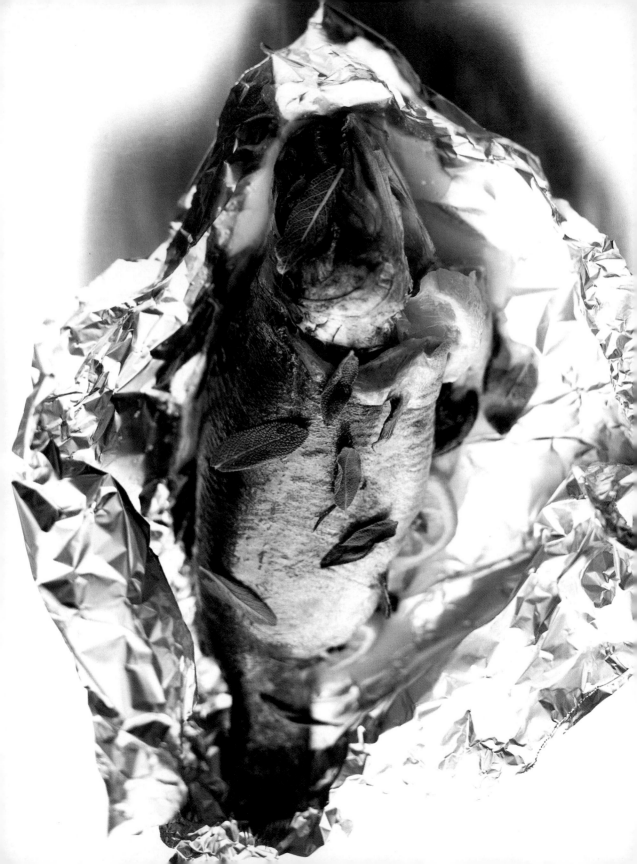

baked salmon with herbs

1	whole salmon or large piece weighing about 2 pounds
½ cup	chopped parsley
2 Tbsp	of any combination of fresh, chopped herbs
1 small	bunch green onions, tops and bottoms trimmed
1 Tbsp	water
1 Tbsp	lemon juice

1. Place salmon on foil. Measure thickest part. Open salmon lengthwise so that you can sprinkle herbs and salt and pepper inside. Lay green onions inside the cavity and close the salmon. Mix water and lemon juice and pour over the outside of the salmon. Fold foil over fish and seal.

2. Place foil-wrapped salmon on a baking sheet and bake in a 450°F oven for 10 minutes for every inch of thickness of fish, plus an additional 10 minutes of cooking time. A total of 45 minutes is usually adequate. Salmon should be opaque but not dry. Unwrap salmon and discard skin, which usually sticks to the foil. Place whole salmon on warmed serving platter and garnish with dill and fresh lemon wedges. Trout can also be used for this recipe.

Makes 4 servings.

PER SERVING
Calories 415
Protein 26 grams
Fat 6 grams
Carbohydrates 1 grams

sautéed baby bok choy

1 cup	low-fat, low-salt chicken broth
¼ tsp	red chili flakes
1	clove garlic, minced
4	baby bok choy

1. Place chicken stock and seasonings in a large frying pan. Over medium heat, bring mixture to a boil.

2. In the meantime, trim the tough ends from bok choy. Rinse and drain.

3. Add bok choy to broth mixture and reduce heat to a simmer. Cook uncovered for about 5 minutes. Using tongs, turn bok choy and continue cooking for another 5 minutes. Drain and serve hot.

Makes 4 servings.

PER SERVING
Calories 26
Protein 3 grams
Fat 0.1 grams
Carbohydrates 3 grams

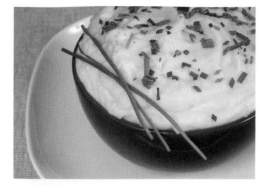

smashed red potatoes

6	red-skinned potatoes, washed and unpeeled
3	cloves garlic, smashed
¼	heated low-fat, sodium-reduced vegetable stock
1 Tbsp	nonfat yogurt
1	green onion, chopped
¼ tsp	each salt, pepper and nutmeg

1 Cut potatoes into 1½-inch chunks. Boil potatoes and garlic in salted water until tender, about 10 -15 minutes. Drain. Place pan on low heat to dry the potatoes, shaking occasionally.

2 Add hot stock and yogurt. Using a potato masher, mash coarsely. The mixture should look lumpy. Stir in the chopped onion and spices.

Makes 4 servings.

PER SERVING
Calories 194
Protein 4 grams
Fat 2 grams
Carbohydrates 39 grams

basic chicken stir-fry

2 small	cloves garlic, minced
2 Tbsp	chopped ginger
3 cups	cooked chicken strips
2 cups	low-fat, low-salt chicken stock
½ cup	snow peas
¼ cup	chopped green onion
½ cup	chopped carrots
½ cup	chopped celery
½ cup	broccoli florets
½ cup	cauliflower florets
¼ cup	red peppers, chopped
2 Tbsp	hoisin sauce
cooking spray	

1. Coat large frying pan or wok with cooking spray. Heat pan or wok over high heat.

2. Stir-fry ginger, garlic and chicken for three minutes or until golden brown.

3. Add all other vegetables and stir-fry until vegetables are tender-crisp. You may need to add a spoonful of water to prevent scorching. Stir in hoisin sauce until mixed.

Makes 4 servings.

PER SERVING
Calories 236
Protein 30 grams
Fat 7 grams
Carbohydrates 14 grams

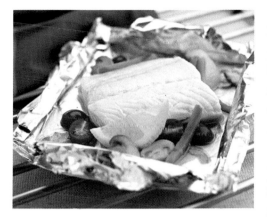

fillet of sole with lemon and parsley

1 pound	sole fillets
Vegetable cooking spray	
1 Tbsp	fresh lemon juice
2 Tbsp	chopped fresh parsley
Salt and pepper	

Place fillets in a baking dish lightly coated with cooking spray. Arrange fish in a single layer. Mist fish lightly with cooking spray. Sprinkle parsley and lemon juice over fish and dust with salt and pepper to taste. Bake uncovered at 450°F until fish is opaque or until it flakes easily.

Makes 4 servings.

PER SERVING
Calories 117
Protein 20 grams
Fat 7 grams
Carbohydrates 1 gram

foil-steamed spring vegetables

¾ pound	fresh baby carrots
½ pound	asparagus
½ pound	small zucchini
1	red pepper
½ pound	snow peas
2 Tbsp	water
1	bay leaf
salt and pepper to taste	

1 In a large pot of boiling water blanch carrots for 2 minutes. Drain and rinse under cold, running water and drain again. Remove tough ends of the asparagus. Top and tail snow peas, and remove fibrous string as well. Wash red pepper and remove seeds and veins. Slice into long pieces about ¼ inch wide.

2 On a large sheet of tin foil, arrange vegetables and sprinkle with water, salt, pepper and bay leaf. Fold foil over vegetables and seal. Bake at 375° F for 20 - 30 minutes or until vegetables are tender.

Makes 6 servings.

PER SERVING
Calories 65
Protein 0.5 grams
Fat 3 grams
Carbohydrates 23 grams

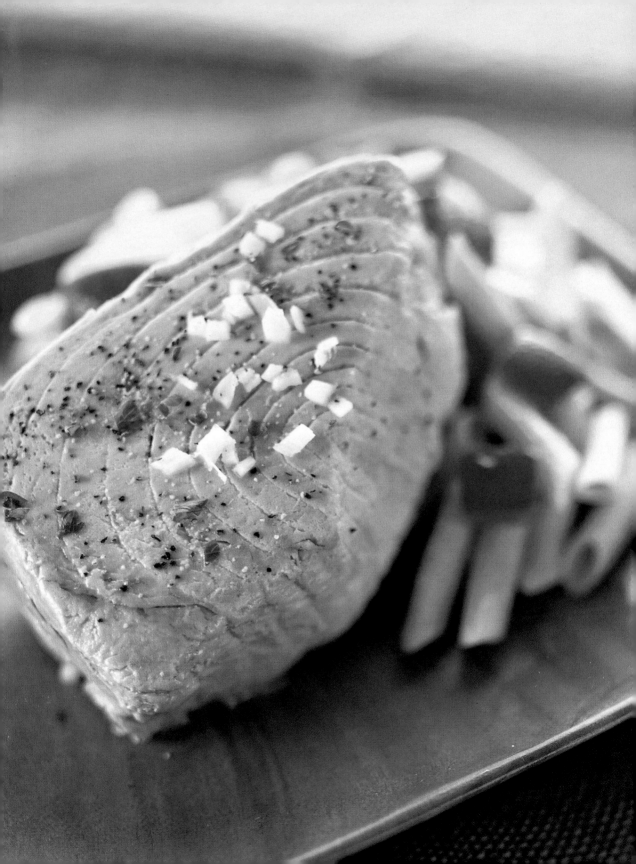

seared tuna

4 (6-ounce)	tuna steaks
8	shiitake or 6 medium-size portobella mushrooms, no stems
10	plum tomatoes, firm and ripe or
4	ripe cluster tomatoes
3 Tbsp	best-quality olive oil
¼ tsp	salt

salt and pepper to taste

1. To make sauce, slice mushrooms into bite-sized strips. Quarter tomatoes. Squeeze juice and tomatoes out of each quarter. Chop remaining tomato flesh. You need about 4 cups.

2. Heat olive oil in large frying pan over medium-high heat. Add mushrooms when oil is very hot. Quickly add ¼ teaspoon salt and stir-fry until mushrooms are lightly browned. Now add tomatoes. Cook over medium heat until mixture is soft and thick.

3. Lightly coat a griddle with cooking spray. Place it over medium-high heat. Sprinkle tuna with salt and pepper. Place in hot frying pan. Sear for 4 minutes each side. Serve with tomato sauce.

Makes 4 servings.

PER SERVING
Calories 452
Protein 45 grams
Fat 24 grams
Carbohydrates 15 grams

stir-fried spinach, asparagus and red onion

1 pound	asparagus
1 small	red onion
1 large	bunch spinach
1 Tbsp	best-quality olive oil
½ tsp	sesame oil
2 cloves	garlic, minced
½ tsp	salt
1 Tbsp	lemon juice or balsamic vinegar

1. Snap tough ends from asparagus. Wash and drain. Slice into two-inch pieces. Slice onion into rings. Trim tough ends from spinach. Wash and drain.

2. Heat olive oil in large frying pan over medium heat.

3. Add onion and garlic. Stir-fry for 4 minutes. Add asparagus and one tablespoon water. Sprinkle with salt. Stir-fry until onion is soft and asparagus is tender-crisp. Add spinach and stir-fry until it's wilted. Stir in lemon juice.

Makes 4 servings.

PER SERVING
Calories 97
Protein 5 grams
Fat 3 grams
Carbohydrates 13 grams

fiesta egg-white scramble

1 Tbsp	extra virgin olive oil
2	green onions, thinly sliced
½	red bell pepper, chopped
1	small tomato, seeded, chopped
1 cup	baby spinach leaves, washed dried and chopped
4	egg whites

salt and freshly ground black pepper to taste

1. Heat oil over medium heat in large frying pan. Add onions, pepper, tomato and spinach and sauté for 3 minutes or until vegetables are soft.

2. Make a well in the center of the vegetables and add eggs. Keeping eggs in the center of the well, stir quickly until egg whites are scrambled.

3. Mix the cooked vegetables into the scrambled eggs. Season with salt and pepper, then serve.

Makes 1 serving.

PER SERVING
Calories 240
Protein 16 grams
Fat 14 grams
Carbohydrates 12 grams

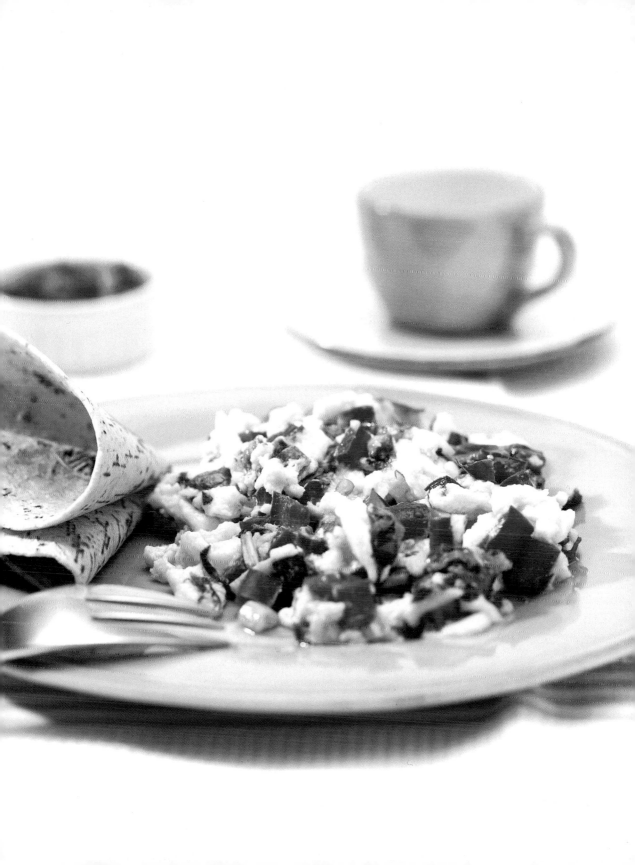

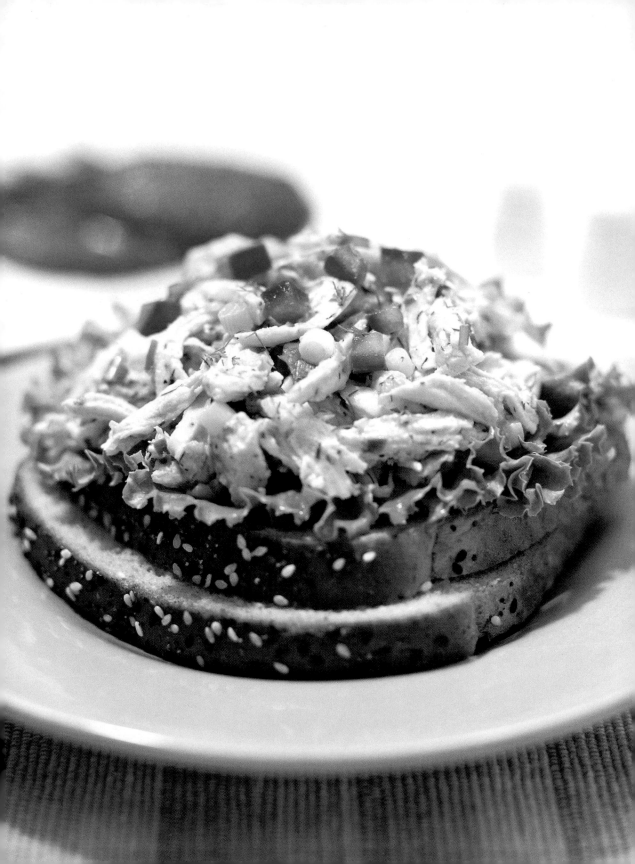

chicken salad sandwich

1 lb	cooked boneless, skinless chicken breast
½ cup	prepared mustard
½ cup	cucumbers, finely chopped
½ cup	scallions, chopped
1 tsp	dill weed seasoning
1 tsp	garlic powder
1 tsp	pepper
12 slices	whole-wheat bread or toast
1	lettuce leaf
2	tomatoes, chopped

1. Shred chicken in a food processor and mix in seasonings. Serve on bread with lettuce and tomato.

Makes 6 servings.

PER SERVING
Calories 318
Protein 26 grams
Fat 7 grams
Carbohydrates 36 grams

great wall steak salad

²/₃ cup	French's Bold'n Spicy Brown Mustard
½ cup	water
¼ cup	reduced-sodium teriyaki sauce
2 Tbsp	fresh ginger, peeled and grated
1 tsp	fresh garlic, minced
1 lb	flank steak, 1-inch thick
8 cups	mixed salad greens, washed and torn
1 medium	yellow or orange bell pepper, thinly sliced
2	green onions, thinly shredded
¼ cup	dry roasted unsalted peanuts

1. In a small bowl, combine mustard, water, teriyaki sauce, ginger and garlic. Set 1 cup of dressing mixture aside.

2. Broil or grill steak for approximately 10 minutes (or until desired tenderness). Baste with the remaining dressing mixture.

3. Let stand for 5 minutes. Place salad greens on 4 plates. Thinly slice steak and evenly divide over greens. Top with bell pepper, onion and peanuts. Drizzel with dressing and serve.

Makes 4 servings.

PER SERVING
Calories 298
Protein 35 grams
Fat 14 grams
Carbohydrates 9 grams

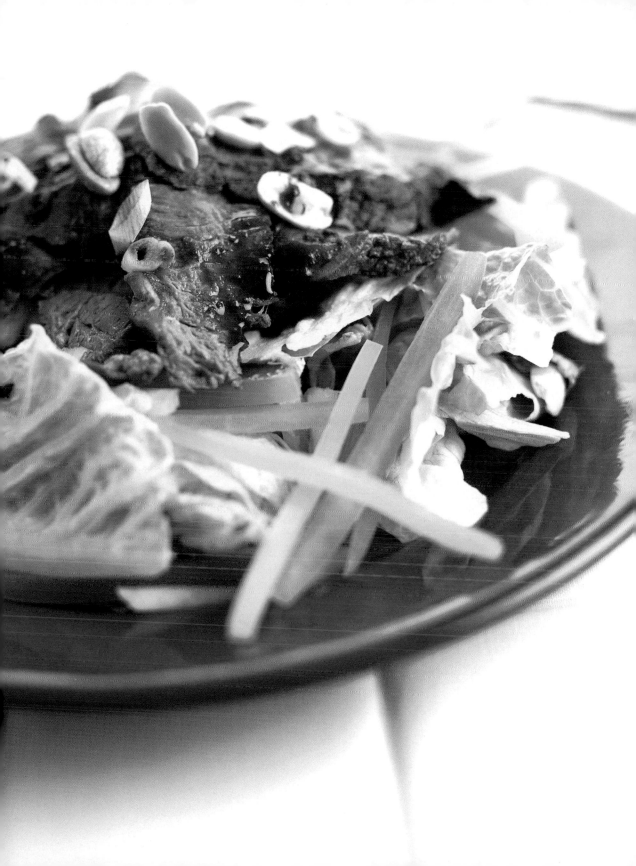

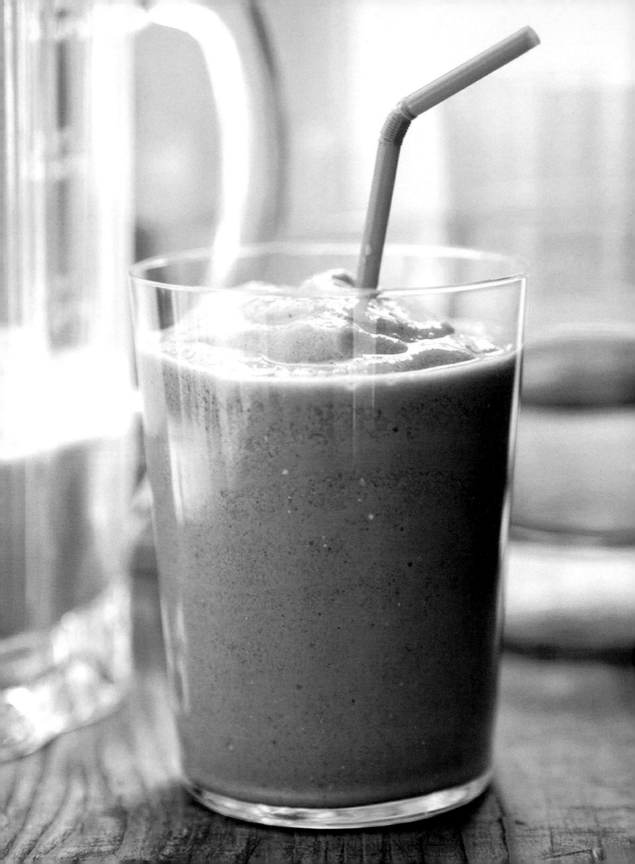

nutty protein smoothie

½ cup	low-fat vanilla soy milk
½ cup	silken tofu
½ cup	water
½ cup	oatmeal
2 Tbsp	natural almond nut butter (or nut butter of your choice)
1 Tbsp	flaxseed
1	banana, peeled
1 cup	ice, crushed

1. Place all ingredients in a blender. Process until smooth. Pour into glass and enjoy.

Makes 1 serving.

PER SERVING
Calories 589
Protein 28 grams
Fat 24 grams
Carbohydrates 69 grams

garlic herbed fish

8 oz	halibut
1	garlic clove, finely chopped
¼ tsp	fresh herbs

1. Cut small slits in top of halibut with a knife and insert garlic and fresh herbs. Double-wrap the fish in plastic wrap and put it in the steamer. Bring water to a boil and cover for eight minutes or until it's done. Serve.

Makes 1 serving.

PER SERVING
Calories 252
Protein 47 grams
Fat 5 grams
Carbohydrates 1 grams

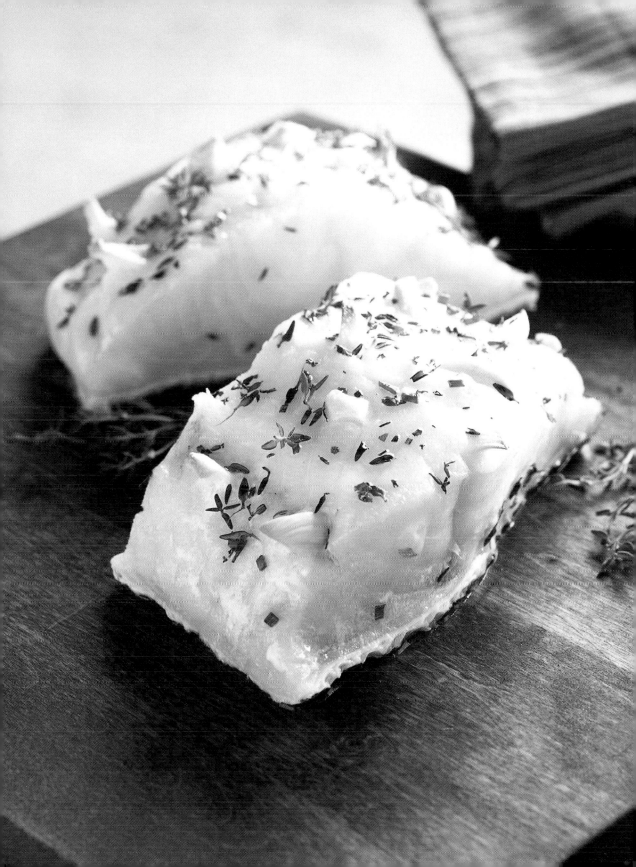

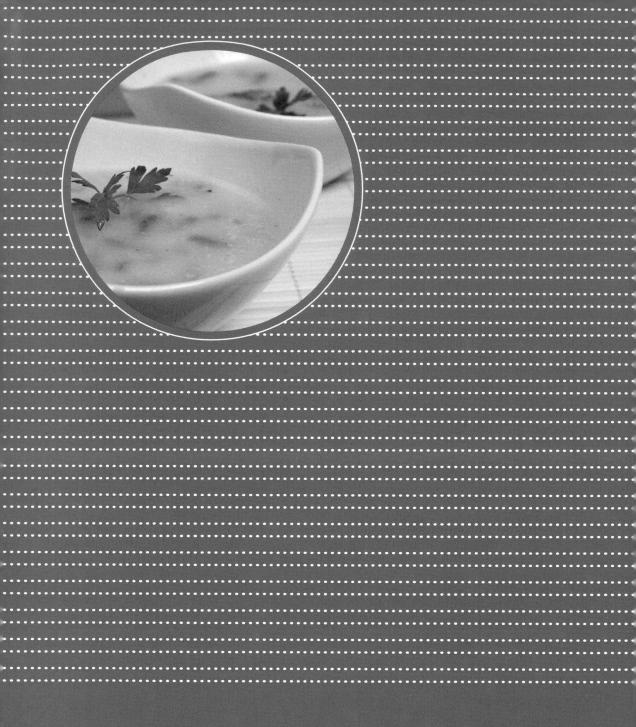

CHAPTER seven

one week of slimming soups

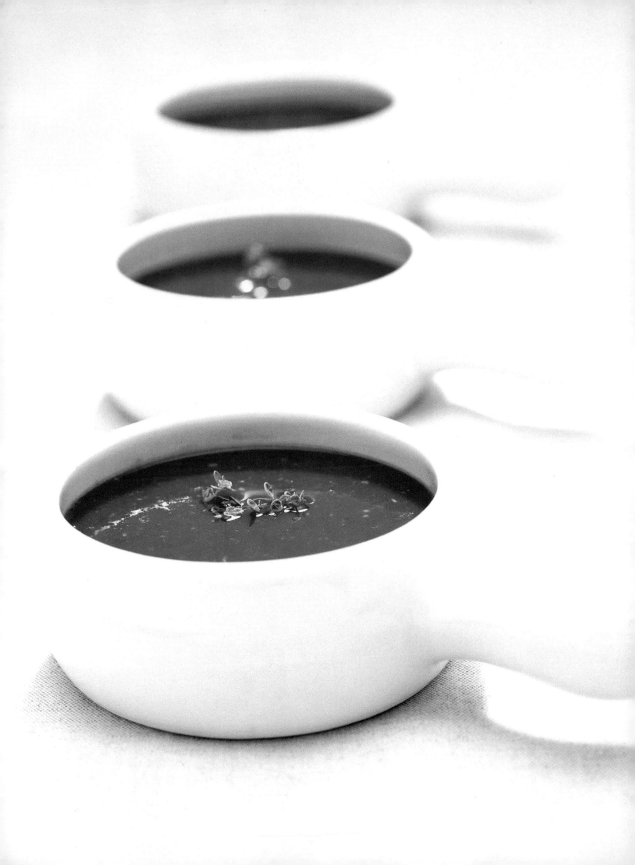

tomato and roasted garlic soup

Roasting garlic in the oven mellows the flavor of this pungent bulb. Garlic contains flavonoids – you know these because flavonoids are responsible for the strong flavor and smell in garlic. The good news is that these smelly chemicals help lower blood pressure, reduce the risk of heart disease and help to fight cancer. When garlic is combined with tomatoes, basil and oregano, it's like eating summer in a bowl, all year long.

1	head garlic
¾ tsp	best-quality olive oil
salt and freshly ground pepper	
1 cup	chopped onion
1 cup	chopped celery
8 cups	stewed tomatoes, including liquid
1	bay leaf
2 tsp	dried basil
1 tsp	dried oregano
1 tsp	dried thyme

1. Preheat oven to 350°F. Remove loose, papery skin from garlic, leaving heads intact. Place garlic on a sheet of heavy-duty foil; drizzle with ¼ teaspoon of olive oil and sprinkle with a pinch of salt and pepper.

2. Loosely wrap foil around garlic, folding edges securely. Roast until garlic has softened, about 40 minutes. Remove from oven and transfer to a plate where it can cool.

3. Open foil carefully and discard. Separate garlic into cloves. Squeeze soft garlic from each clove into a small bowl. Set aside.

4. In a large saucepan over medium heat allow remaining ½ teaspoon olive oil to heat. Add onion, celery and roasted garlic. Cover and cook until vegetables soften, about 5 minutes. Stir in tomatoes, 1 cup water, bay leaf, basil, oregano, thyme and ¼ teaspoon pepper. Bring mixture to a boil. Reduce heat and simmer for a further 15 minutes, allowing time to blend flavors.

5. Using a hand blender, purée the soup until mostly smooth.

Makes about 6 servings.

PER SERVING
Calories 113
Protein 3 grams
Fat 2 grams
Carbohydrates 23 grams

DAY TWO

spa vegetable soup

Keep low-fat, low-sodium chicken stock on hand in your pantry to make this quick and easy soup. Just add an interesting array of chopped vegetables to make a delicious and low-fat soup for lunch or dinner.

3 cups	low-fat, low-sodium chicken stock
1	carrot, peeled and diagonally sliced
1 cup	celery, diagonally sliced
½ cup	finely sliced savoy cabbage, red cabbage or spinach
1 cup	cauliflower florets
1 cup	broccoli florets
1	green onion, diagonally sliced

salt and pepper to taste

1. In a saucepan, bring chicken stock to a boil. Add carrot and simmer for 10 minutes.

2. Add remaining vegetables and simmer until tender, about 15 minutes.

3. Season with salt and pepper to taste.

Makes 4 servings.

PER SERVING
Calories 27
Protein 2 grams
Fat 0.5 grams
Carbohydrates 4 grams

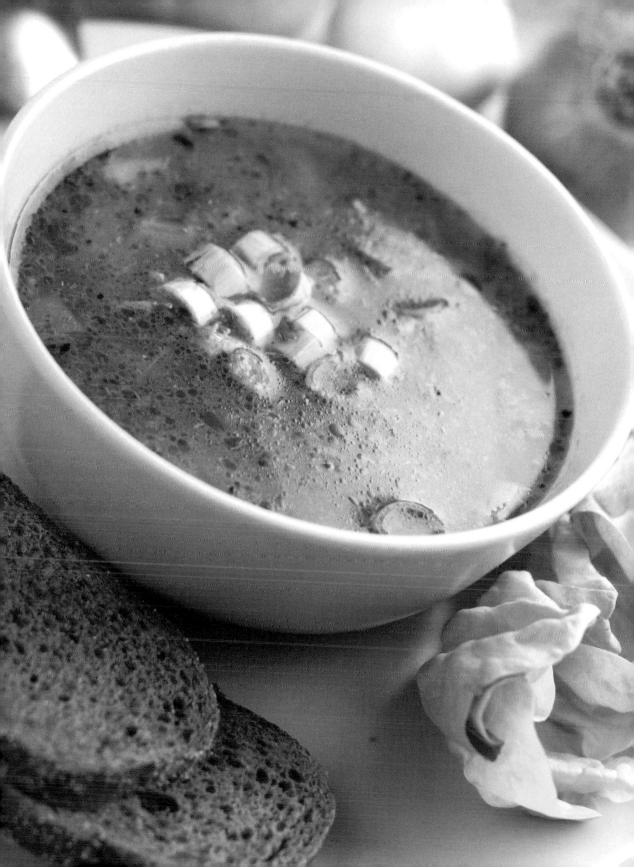

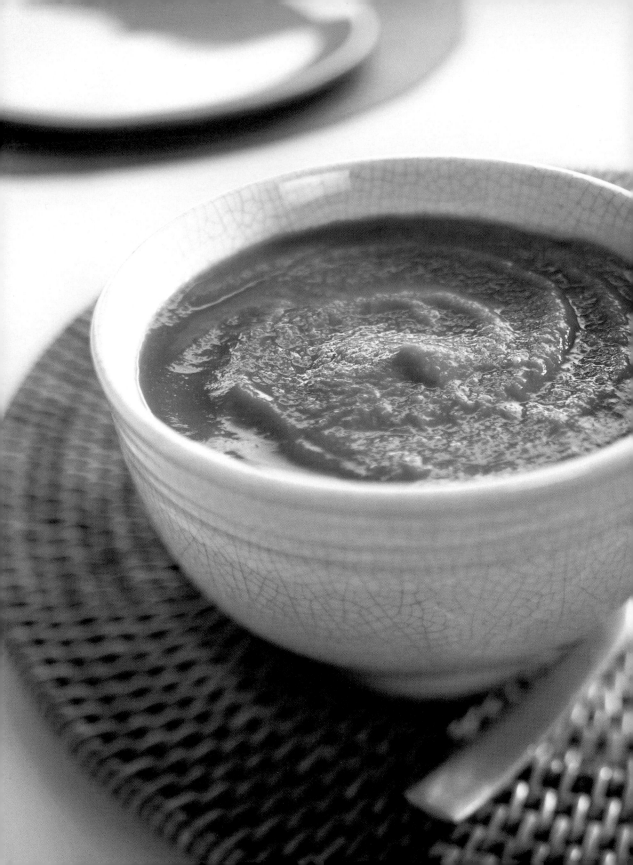

DAY THREE

curried pumpkin soup

1 Tbsp	olive oil
1	onion, chopped
1	clove garlic, minced
2 tsp	curry powder
1 tsp	cumin
½ tsp	cayenne
3	apples, peeled, cored and chopped
15-oz	can pumpkin puree
2 ⅔ cups low-sodium chicken broth
⅔ cup	water
1 tsp	white sugar

1. Pour oil into a large saucepan and place over medium heat. Add onion, garlic, curry powder, cumin and cayenne.

2. Sauté, stirring often, until onion is soft. Stir in apples, pumpkin, broth, water, and sugar.

3. Bring to a boil, cover, and reduce heat to low. Simmer for 25 minutes, stirring occasionally.

4. Purée soup in a food processor or blender. Just before serving, return to pot on low heat.

Makes 6 servings.

PER SERVING
Calories 93
Protein 1 grams
Fat 3 grams
Carbohydrates 15.5 grams

DAY FOUR

white bean and collard green soup

A member of the kale family, collard greens are packed with calcium. When combined with onions, garlic and beans, this easy soup is a nutritional giant. Studies show that consuming these foods can reduce the risk of heart disease. Try using kale if you can't find collard greens.

2 Tbsp	best-quality olive oil
2 cups	chopped onion
3 Tbsp	garlic, finely chopped
1	bay leaf
3 or 4	stalks celery, chopped
2	thick carrots, peeled and chopped
1 tsp	salt
6 cups	low-fat, low-sodium chicken stock
4 cups	cooked white beans
1 bunch	collard greens, well washed, chopped and stemmed
4	grilled, skinless chicken breasts, diced – *optional*

salt and pepper to taste

1. In a stockpot, heat olive oil over medium-low heat. Add onion, bay leaf, celery and carrots. Cook over low heat for about 10 minutes or until vegetables are soft.

2. Add stock. Cover and bring mixture to a boil. Reduce heat and simmer for 20 minutes or until vegetables are tender.

3. Add white beans, garlic and collard greens or kale. Cover. In about 15 to 20 minutes the leafy vegetables will have softened enough to allow blending.

4. Add salt and pepper to taste.

Makes 4 to 6 servings.

PER SERVING *(with chicken)*
Calories 326
Protein 27 grams
Fat 7 grams
Carbohydrates 41 grams

PER SERVING *(without chicken)*
Calories 260
Protein 13 grams
Fat 6 grams
Carbohydrates 40 grams

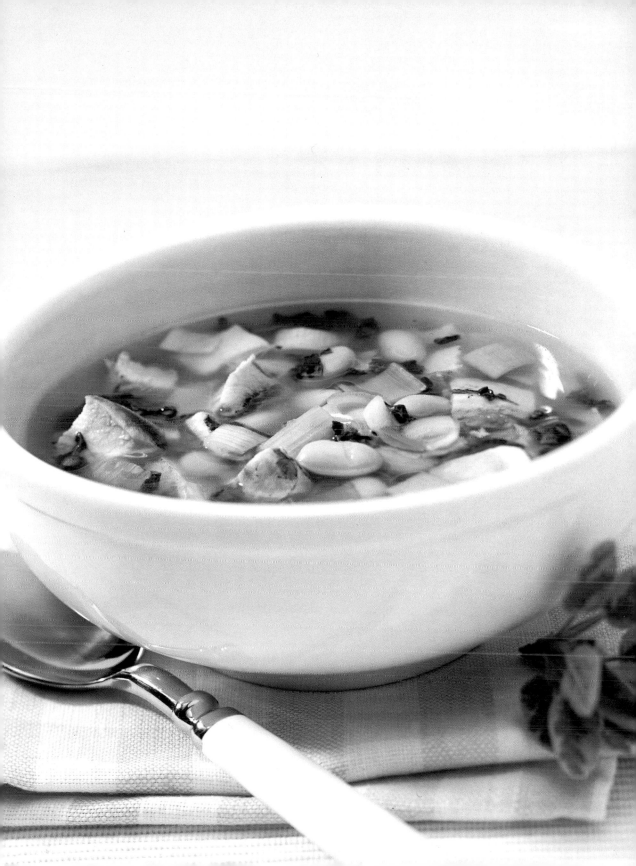

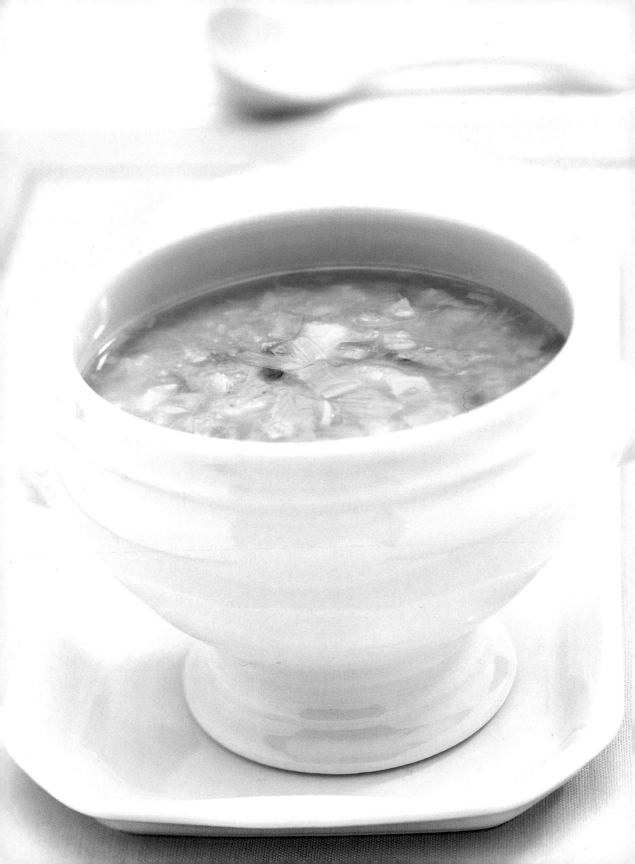

leek, potato and herb soup

A wonderful variation to leek and potato soup, this soup is chunkier and heartier. Known to cleanse the blood, leeks and asparagus combine to make a thick and healthy soup.

1 Tbsp	best-quality olive oil
2	medium leeks, whites only, washed and chopped
2	garlic cloves, minced
4 or 5	new potatoes, washed and cubed
4 cups	low-fat, low-sodium chicken stock
1 cup	zucchini, chopped
1 cup	asparagus, chopped
1 Tbsp	parsley, chopped
2 Tbsp	chives, chopped
salt and pepper to taste	

1. Heat olive oil in a large soup kettle and add leeks. Cook over medium-low heat until softened, about 5 minutes.

2. Add garlic and cook for a few minutes.

3. Now add the stock and potatoes. Bring to a boil and reduce heat to medium. Simmer vegetables for 20 minutes until soft.

4. Add zucchini and asparagus. Cook for 10 minutes.

5. Remove soup pot from heat. Add chopped herbs.

6. Using a hand blender, blend the soup until it reaches desired consistency.

Makes 4 servings.

PER SERVING
Calories 157
Protein 5 grams
Fat 5 grams
Carbohydrates 25 grams

DAY SIX

squash soup health purée

Squash becomes plentiful during the fall and winter months. With its vibrant colors and meaty texture, it makes an excellent base for hearty soups. Squash also works well with pumpkin pie spices like cinnamon and allspice. Bursting with free-radical-fighting antioxidants, squash is a must in your clean-eating regimen.

8 cups	low-fat, low-sodium chicken stock
6 cups	coarsely chopped, peeled winter squash
1	onion, cut into chunks
3 large	garlic cloves, minced
2	carrots, peeled and cut into chunks
1	red bell pepper, seeded and chopped
2	sweet potatoes, peeled and chopped
2	parsnips, peeled and cut into chunks
2 tsp	cinnamon
¼ tsp	allspice
salt and pepper to taste	

1. Place chicken stock in large soup kettle and bring to a boil.

2. Reduce heat and add all vegetables, garlic and spices. Simmer until all vegetables are tender, about 30 minutes.

3. Using a hand blender or food processor, purée soup.

4. Season with salt and pepper.

Makes 6 servings.

PER SERVING
Calories 137
Protein 4 grams
Fat 1 grams
Carbohydrates 31 grams

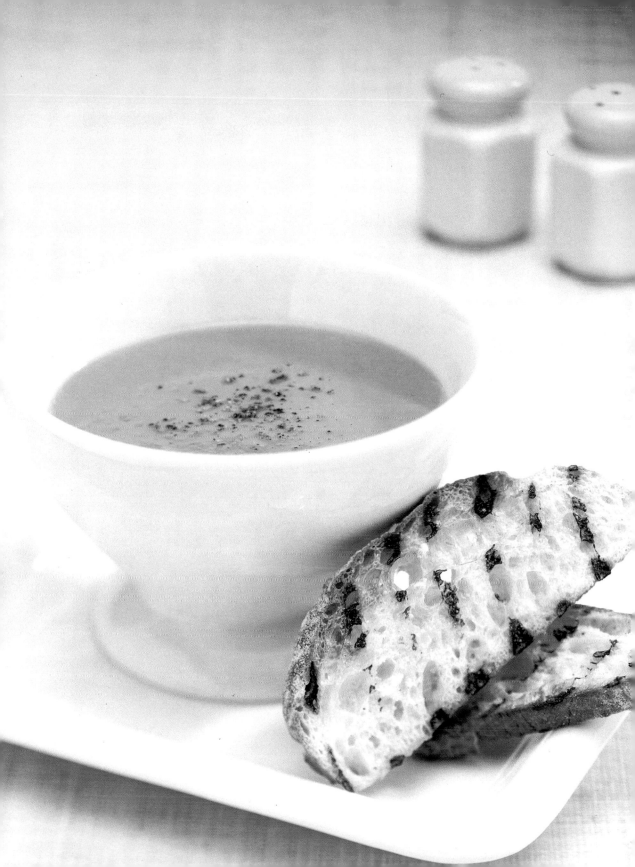

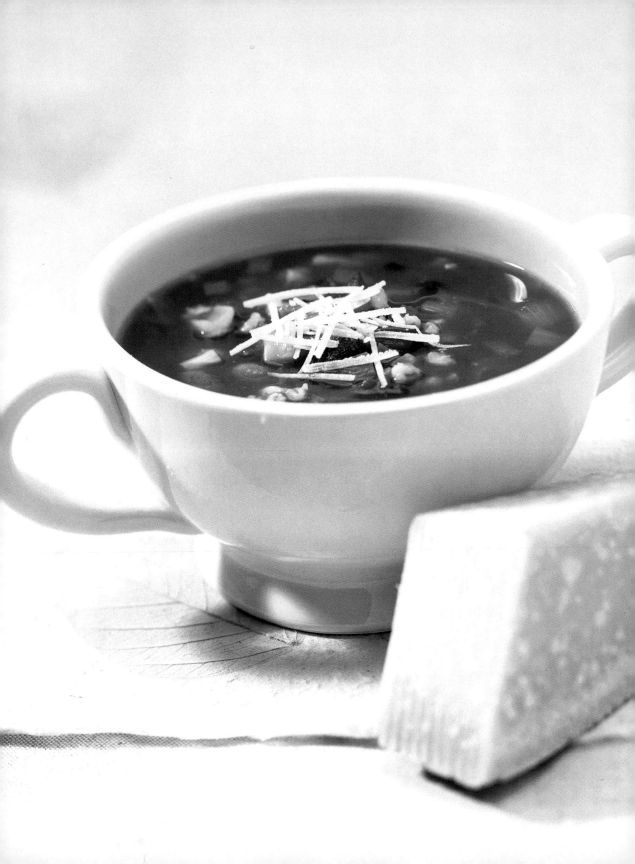

bean, potato and red pepper soup

This robust soup contains protein and complex carbohydrates for a nutritionally balanced main course with staying power. Just add a slice of hearty, whole-grain bread and you have an easy, nourishing meal. Take leftovers for lunch.

3 cups	canned navy beans, drained and rinsed
8 cups	low-fat, low-sodium chicken stock
4 large	potatoes, peeled and cubed
1	bay leaf
2 Tbsp	best-quality olive oil
2 cups	diced onion
2 cups	diced celery
2 cups	diced carrots
3 large	garlic cloves, minced
2 red	bell peppers, seeded and diced
6 cups	crushed tomatoes, with liquid
Salt and pepper to taste	

1. In large soup kettle, bring stock to a boil. Add beans, potatoes and bay leaf. Simmer until tender, about 30 minutes.

2. In large skillet, heat olive oil. Add onion, celery, carrots and garlic. Sautée until soft. Add to soup.

3. Stir in red peppers and tomatoes and simmer for another 15 minutes.

4. Using a hand blender, purée soup until smooth.

5. Season with salt and pepper.

Makes 6 servings.

PER SERVING
Calories 486
Protein 19 grams
Fat 7 grams
Carbohydrates 94 grams

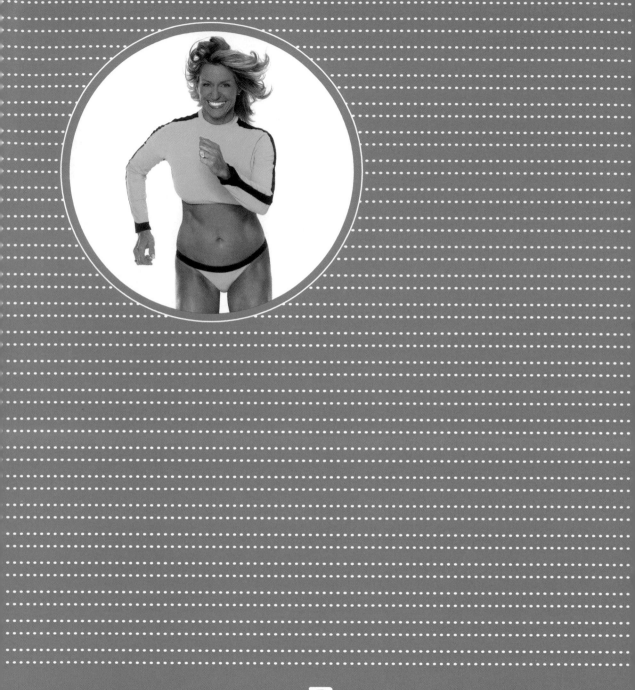

CHAPTER eight

33 tips for your best butt ever!

1. Get Real – Get Naked
2. Check-up
3. Runway Butt, Not!
4. Junk Food
5. Form
6. Gym Wear
7. Goal Setting
8. Read Up on the Subject
9. Visualization
10. Inspiration
11. Sets and Reps
12. Embarrassment
13. Keep the Muscles Surprised
14. No Weighing
15. Rest Time
16. Record Keeping
17. Diet
18. Flush Out Your System
19. Mind To Muscle
20. Squeeze
21. Complete Training
22. Frequency
23. Specific Butt Training
24. Squeeze Walking
25. Love Your Butt
26. Magazines
27. Breathing
28. Sugar
29. Mental Focus
30. Fallacy
31. Intensity
32. All-Round Training
33. No Gym

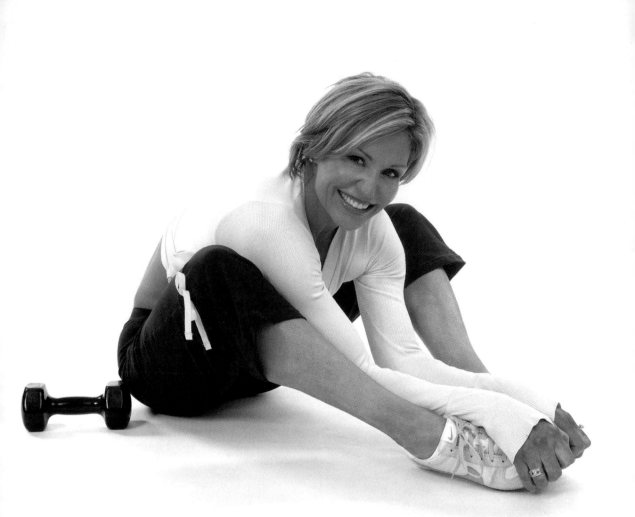

Whatever the present condition of your glutes right now, believe me, they can be improved beyond your wildest dreams from day one. Follow these 33 tips and enjoy the ecstasy of a perfectly formed derriere. Don't just read and turn the page – read and act. It is your pro-active approach to following these suggestions that will give you the magic shape and condition you desire ...

Let me know of your success!

1 get real – get naked

Check yourself out in the mirror. Don't look for the most favorable light. This is the time for honest self-evaluation. Re-assess yourself on a regular basis.

check-up

Before starting a new diet or exercise regimen get an okay from your family physician. Ask to have a physical stress test. This advice is essential, especially if you are a heavy smoker or over 40.

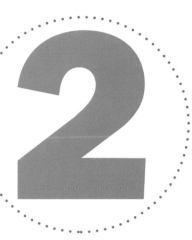

3. **runway butt, not!**

Banish from your mind the preconceived notion that a high-fashion runway model's flat butt is the ideal for womankind. The truly fit butt is curvaceous and toned, not flat and soft.

4 junk food

Your backside will mirror what you ingest – cookies, doughnuts and ice cream will give you a soft, spongy, sugar-candy tush.

form

Use sufficient resistance when training glutes, but maintain perfect form throughout. A sloppy technique will not build a tight tush.

6. gym wear

Wear loose-fitting gym apparel when exercising. Tight Versace jeans are not the way to go. *Comfort is the name of the game.*

7 goal setting

Set believable goals. Plan for changes every four to six weeks. Once you reach your goal, set another. It has to be realistic.

read up on the subject 8

Call toll free 1-888-254-0767 to order *The Bottom Line*, by Robert Kennedy.

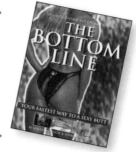

9. **visualization**

Visualize yourself as lean and mean, not soft and fat. With proper focus on visualization your physique will follow suit.

10 inspiration

Find a photograph of what you consider to be the perfect posterior and place it on your fridge or bathroom mirror.

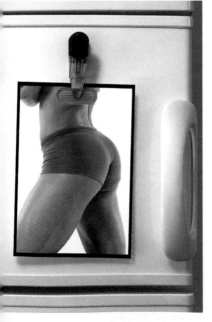

11. sets and reps

Low reps should not be part of your glute training. Keep the reps higher than twelve, but only occasionally go over twenty. Sets should number from two to four for each movement, depending on your energy levels, age and present level of fitness.

12 embarrassment

Ignore the glances of others. Your derriere may not be perfect now, but you will succeed. Use the humiliation you feel to keep your training enthusiasm at a constant high. In time, embarrassment will turn to pride. Hang in there.

13. keep the muscles surprised

Work out using at least three butt-specific movements each glute-training day. Drop one and substitute a different glute exercise every few workouts. Rotating your butt exercises in this way will keep your butt tight.

14 no weighing

Throw out your scales. Muscle weighs more than fat. Let the mirror and only the mirror be your guide. Your actual weight is inconsequential.

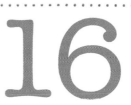

15. **rest time**

Rest 45 to 60 seconds between sets. A specialized butt workout should be completed in about 15 minutes.

record keeping

Keep a record of what sets, reps and weight resistance you use each training session. *Oxygen's* training journal is available by calling toll free 1-888-254-0767.

16

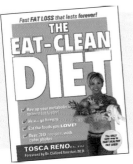
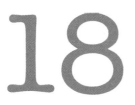

17. diet

Clean up your nutrition. Base your diet around grilled chicken, fish, veggies, berries, egg whites, rice, sweet potatoes and oatmeal. Never underestimate the vital importance of diet in shaping your backside. Order **The Eat-Clean Diet** at **1-866-837-6032** or go online to **www.eatcleandiet.com**.

18 flush out your system

Drink water throughout the day. Toxins love to collect in fat, which can lead to cellulite accumulation. Water drinking helps your body process to function at top level. The book *Water*, by Patricia Bragg, is extremely informative. Check it out at www.bragg.com.

19. mind to muscle

Mentally place the action into the glutes while training. Occasionally touch your glute muscles while exercising to help put your mind and focus into the muscle.

20 squeeze

Contract and squeeze your butt muscles while you perform each glute-specific repetition. The idea is to exhaust the glutes as quickly as possible.

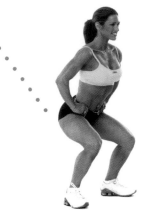

21. complete training

Make a point of hitting all three areas of the glutes. The high part, the middle and lower areas. The butt is a workhorse and can take a good deal of punishment. Learn to love the burn and tailor your exercises to your immediate needs.

22. frequency

Train the glutes two times a week, making sure that you have at least two non-glute training days between sessions.

23. specific butt training

Recognizing glute training as part of your exercise regimen. You will not build rock-hard glutes with shoulder presses, curls or even cardio. Specific butt exercises are required.

24 squeeze walking

Tighten your glutes each stride while going for a country walk or hike. However, doing this in your local mall could get you some weird looks.

25. love your butt

Clothes look great on a well-rounded, tight backside. Learn to love your butt as a muscle. The glutes are not genitalia. They are pure muscle. Be proud of their shape and rotundity.

26 magazines

Keep up to date with your reading. *Oxygen* magazine (women's fitness) has tons of articles on shaping your butt (and the rest of your body, too). Order online at www.oxygenmag.com or call 1-800-946-5349.

27. breathing

Oxygenate the body by breathing deeply while exercising or walking – fresh air and exercise helps keep fat at bay.

28. **sugar**

Go natural. Avoid sugar and sugar-loaded food products. The body processes sugar by dumping extra fat on the hips, thighs and butt.

29. mental focus

Instead of would-have, should-have, could-have, adopt a positive mental attitude. Whatever you look like now, believe in yourself. Say "yes I can!" Never give up the battle.

30 fallacy

Don't believe for one minute that specialized glute exercises will give you an oversized butt. Regular progressive resistance exercise (weight training) is magical. It will build up an undersized flat butt and shape up, trim and tighten an oversized butt.

31. intensity

Endeavor to increase intensity every few workouts. This is accomplished by increasing reps, adding weight or decreasing rest time between sets. Aim for only small increases. Jumping up in reps or resistance too rapidly will cause you to lose form and could lead to overtraining.

32. all-round training

Do not neglect other body parts. It makes no sense to only exercise your glutes. Devote some exercise time to your torso and limbs. Leg work in particular compliments your glute-training program. They can often be trained together. Suggested reading: *Body Fitness for Women* ($24.95). Order toll free at 1-888-254-0767.

no gym

If you can't get to the gym and have no apparatus at home you can still give your butt a good workout. Many exercises do not require special apparatus. Freestanding squats, lying hip thrusts, squeeze walking, stair climbing, standing kickbacks and lunges all work the glutes.

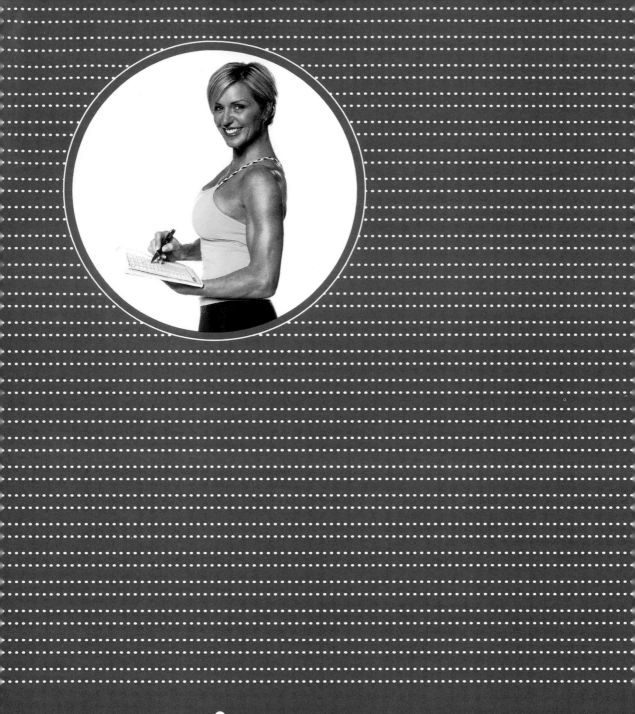

questions &
answers

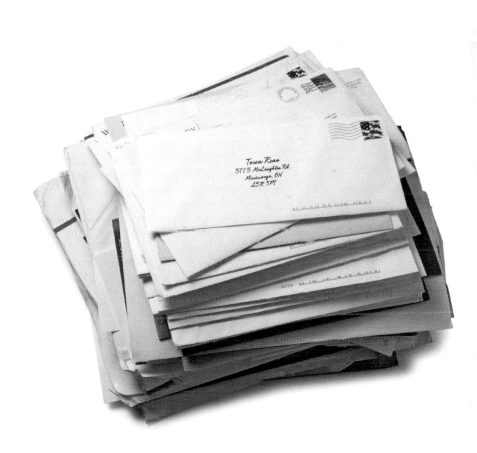

What part do anabolic steroids play in glute development?

Many athletes, bodybuilders and pro sports people of both sexes take anabolic steroids. It is true that steroids, mainly composed of synthetic testosterone compounds, greatly contribute to added hardness of the physique. They also have a tendency to chase fat away. Both effects make the glutes look more round and attractively curved. But there is no question that steroids are seriously harmful to your health. They are not recommended. What kind of harm do they cause? They contribute to hardening of the blood vessels and cause damage to the kidneys, liver and heart. They increase the likelihood of cancer and leukemia. Further reasons not to get involved with these potent drugs are the undesirable side effects of increased facial hair, loss of hair on the head, deepening of the voice, clitoral enlargement and hardening of facial features.

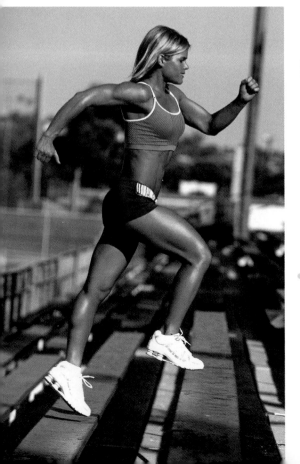

I just do not want to go to the gym. But I do want to exercise and get great buns. Are there any house-friendly glute exercises you can recommend?

This book has a chapter on non-apparatus glute training. Climbing stairs is also an extremely good butt-shaping exercise. Climbing stairs two at a time is even better. People who walk a lot can work their glute area effectively by strongly squeezing each butt cheek as they push back with their legs as they take a step. With practice this can be done without anyone noticing.

Is it really necessary to eat every few hours to develop my glutes?

Your glutes are muscles and muscles are built from protein. It is important that you include a high-protein item with every meal and that you eat every two or three hours. This is not carved-in-stone advice but it is the preferred way to eat if you are serious about fitness. Best protein foods include lean meats, fish, poultry, skim milk, low-fat cheese, egg whites, fat-free yogurt and unsalted nuts. Good carb items that go hand in hand with your high-protein foods include all vegetables, sweet potatoes, salads without dressing, whole-grain breads, oatmeal, fruits and brown rice.

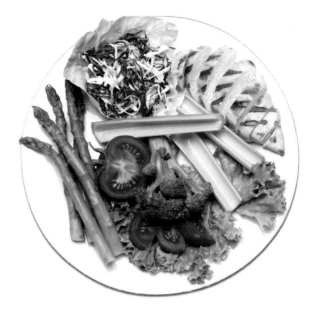

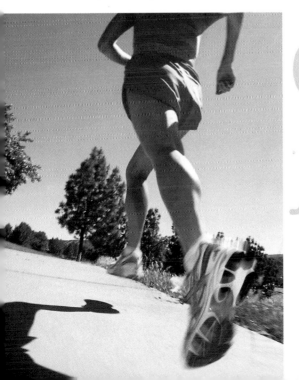

Do athletics contribute to the shaping and development of the backside?

Yes, definitely. Most athletics involve the entire body. Naturally some work the butt more than others. A competitive sprinter or speed skater will build a better butt than a swimmer or a long-distance runner. Generally speaking, all sports contribute to toning the backside and reducing body-fat levels, both of which add to ultimate butt perfection.

How many times a week should I train my backside?

Train your butt once, twice or three times a week. There isn't much difference. Most people find they achieve the best results from two training sessions per week. If you are currently overweight in the butt area it may be a good idea to train your backside more frequently. In addition you should perform higher than normal repetitions – as many as fifteen to twenty-five.

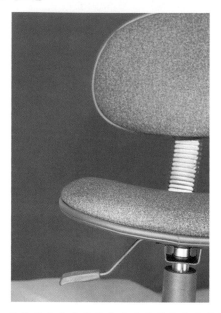

I sit down all day at the office and spend the rest of my time in a car. Will this give me a flat backside?

No. You will, however, get a flat, shapeless backside if you don't exercise and if you eat junk food. If you train regularly your backside will not be negatively affected by sitting down at your office job or driving your car.

I have a treadmill at home. Will this allow me enough exercise to give me perfect glutes?

No. However you can really work the glutes on the treadmill by setting the speed at a very low rate and consciously pushing back with each leg, deliberately tensing the glute muscle as you do so. This is a method that WWE wrestling star, Trish Stratus, uses to keep her buns high, rounded and rock hard.

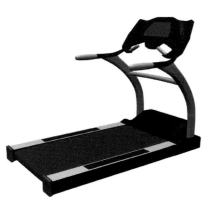

Q: I am confused. There is so much talk about J. Lo's butt and other bottoms like that of Molly Sims. What's up with this?

J. Lo's butt is genetically high and rounded. She varies her body weight greatly and at times has a very healthy looking ghetto-booty while at other times she has a smaller backside, which comes about from a reduced overall bodyweight. Whatever her weight, the butt is still there, curved and high. Molly Sims is a swimsuit and lingerie model who doesn't have a butt. This is in line with the high-fashion, runway model image of flat butts. This book is not about how to get a flat butt. On the contrary, we want to impart everything known about how to build a curvaceous, high, rounded and rock-hard butt.

Q: I want to have a rock-hard, rounded glutes that would stop bullets. But I am confused about how to exercise the rest of my body.

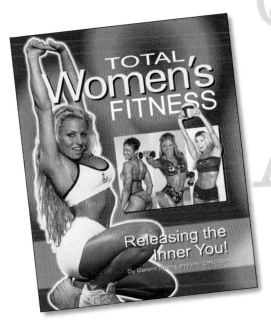

You have asked a good question. Although this book is primarily concerned with glute building and shaping, it is not a good idea to exercise only the glutes. One needs all-round exercise that works every part of the body. The book *Total Women's Fitness* by Gerard Thorne and Phil Embleton will teach you everything you need to know about complete body training. This book is available at Borders bookstores or can be ordered online at www.amazon.com. Alternatively you can order it by calling the following 24/7 toll-free order line. Have your credit card handy. 1-888-254-0767.

What part do genetics play in the shape and hardness of a backside?

Genetics do play an important role. It is not politically correct to single out the natural physical traits of people in different areas of the world but political correctness is not high on my list of priorities at this moment. I am here to help you build a perfect backside. Period. It is obvious that butt shape tends (I said tends, not always), to fall in line with the characteristics of various cultures and races. North American Natives, Asians and East Indians tend to have flatter rear ends, while Africans and African Americans often have backsides that stand out, with high, rounded curves. Europeans seem to fall somewhere in between.

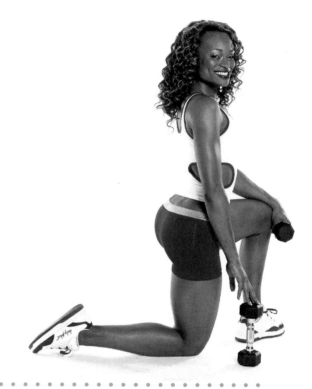

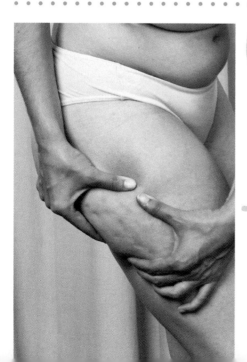

I have cellulite on my backside. Would it help if I exfoliate my skin? What can I do to get rid of this condition?

It is not a bad idea to exfoliate the entire body, including the backside. However, cellulite problems lie deep under and inside the skin's membranes. Cellulite is caused by a junk-food diet and inactivity. You need to eat a clean diet, exercise vigorously and get plenty of fresh air and rest.

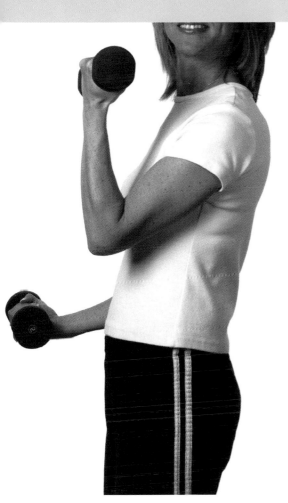

I am over sixty years old. My butt is flat and devoid of curves. Is there anything I can do about this?

A sixty-year-old butt is not going to be as rounded as that of a twenty-year-old. Sensible exercise as described in this book will help greatly, but results will not be sensational. At your age you should make sure that you have a tolerance for strenuous exercise. It is advised that you get an okay from your family physician before starting any new exercise or diet program. Ask for a physical exam and stress test. Chances are you will be given an enthusiastic go ahead, but it is always wise to make sure you are fit enough to take on something new.

From the front or back I almost seem to have a double rear-end. It's rounded at the hips, then rounded again at the bottom where my butt meets my thighs. Am I stuck with this shape?

You tend to collect fat at the two points you mention, and because you have little muscle tone you lose any shape in between. A clean diet and butt-shaping exercise program will work miracles for you. If you work on building up your glutes – remember, they are muscles! – and reducing your body-fat level, you will discover a radically new buttock shape.

Q I'm not that overweight but I probably need to lose 15 pounds to get the butt I want. The trouble is my husband. He insists on keeping chocolate, potato chips and beer in the house and then convinces me to share them with him. What can I do?

A It can be difficult when our loved ones undermine our plans. Of course the best scenario would be to convince him that he should clean up his diet. At the very least, sit down with him and explain how important it is to you that you reach your goal. Let him know that it doesn't make you feel good to ingest these items – rather it makes you feel bad. Enlist his help. Tell him if he absolutely must eat these products to please keep them away from you and preferably out of the house altogether. Once he loses his partner in crime he may lose the taste for this garbage himself. Best of luck.

Q Every woman in my family (including me) has a huge backside. I'm slim, with a 26-inch waist, but my hip measurement is 42 inches! Not only do I look bad, it's really hard to find clothes. Is there anything I can do about this?

A There is no question that genetics play a part in body shape, but I'll say it again: If you keep a clean diet, perform cardio regularly and do the butt exercises laid out in this book you will vastly improve the look of your posterior. There is nothing wrong with having a big rear-end, as long as it's firm and shapely instead of jiggly and saggy. In fact, many men find a big derriere a distinct turn-on.

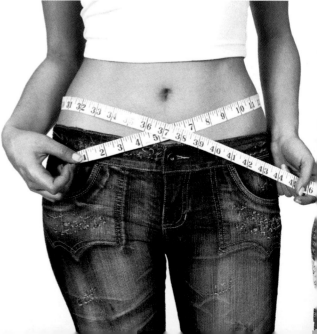

I don't understand why I should go through all this trouble to get a high, round backside when all I really have to do is get implants.

Well, if you have a few thousand dollars burning a hole in your wallet, if you don't mind the possible complications that go with any surgery, if you don't mind the risk of the implant rupturing and you don't mind that the rest of your body will still be flabby and sagging, then go for it! However, if you want long-lasting results that make not just your butt, but also your legs, abs, arms and back look fantastic, and if you want to have glowing skin, lustrous hair and tons of energy to go along with that great body, you'll go with our easy-to-follow program, instead.

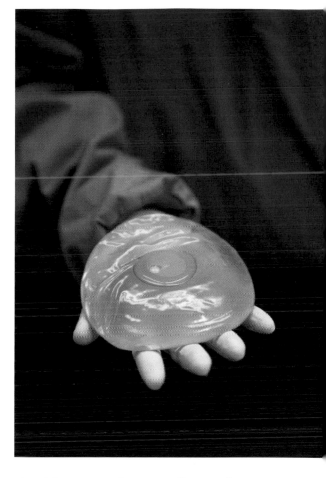

Is it better to just select one butt exercise and work it hard for 4 or 5 sets or is there an advantage to selecting a variety of exercises and doing a couple of sets of each?

Both systems work. If you select just one butt exercise you had better make sure it's a real good one. My suggestion is that you choose the kneeling low-cable kickback on a bench. If really does hit all areas of the derriere. Why not alternate? Try keeping to just one exercise for a month for six sets each workout, and for the following month you can select three different exercises and perform two or three sets each. The variety will keep things progressing.

Q I have a totally non-existent behind. My boyfriend really likes buxom butts, but what can I do? I'm as flat as a pancake!

A You need more food, especially protein. Make sure you eat six times a day. Every meal should contain some complex carbs (veggies, whole grains, sweet potatoes) and protein (grilled skinless chicken, water-packed tuna, egg-white omelet). Relaxation is important to muscle building, as is sound sleep – a minimum of seven hours a night.

Keep up the weight training. The best butt-mass builder is the back squat. Go for three or four sets of twelve reps each leg workout.

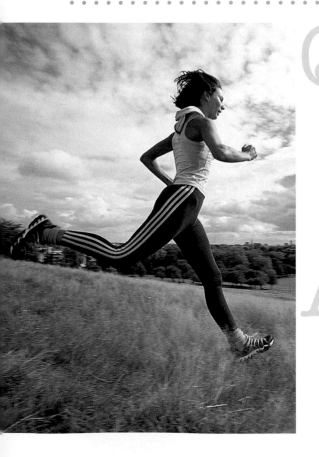

Q I like long-distance running. It keeps my weight down and my muscles toned. However, I'm concerned about my lack of butt roundness. Is there something about running that keeps me from having rounded glutes?

A It depends on whether one is a sprinter or a long-distance runner. Sprinters usually have very well-developed glutes. Long-distance runners are invariably light framed or even downright skinny, and therefore have non-existent butts. If you were to take up sprinting you would be certain to improve your butt contour. The choice is yours.

I just had a baby. I knew that my stomach wouldn't look like it used to, but I had no idea my behind would get all out of shape, too! Just 'cause I'm a mother doesn't mean I don't want to look sexy anymore. What can I do?

Breastfeeding really helps a woman get back into shape, but of course you need diet and exercise too. For the first couple of months stick to lighter exercises that don't put too much pressure on your pelvic area ... it's been through a lot and needs some time to heal. Walking is a great exercise, and you can certainly practice the butt squeeze! You can also do any of the non-apparatus glute exercises in chapter 2. After the first couple of months you can start adding some weights. Eat clean for you and your baby and after a few months you should have your old body back.

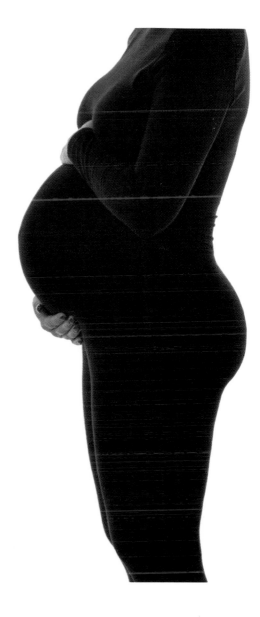

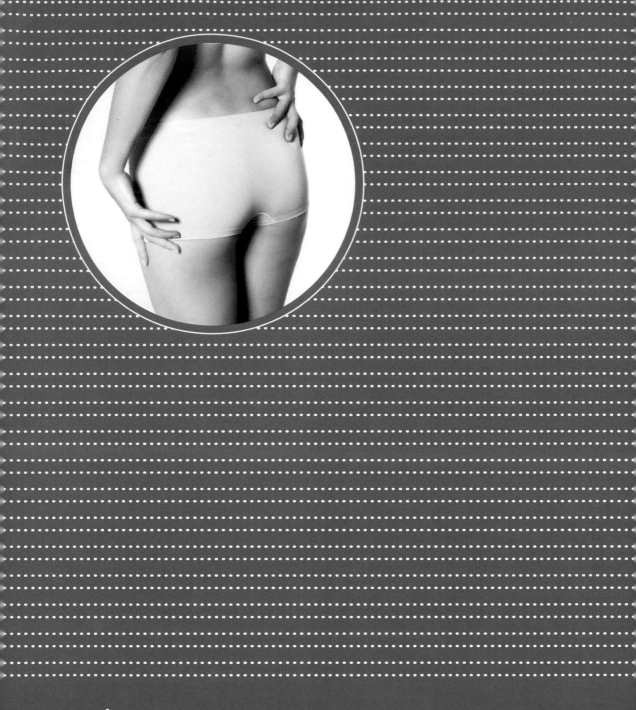

CHAPTER ten

the bodyweight factor

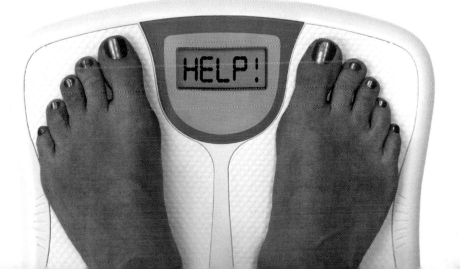

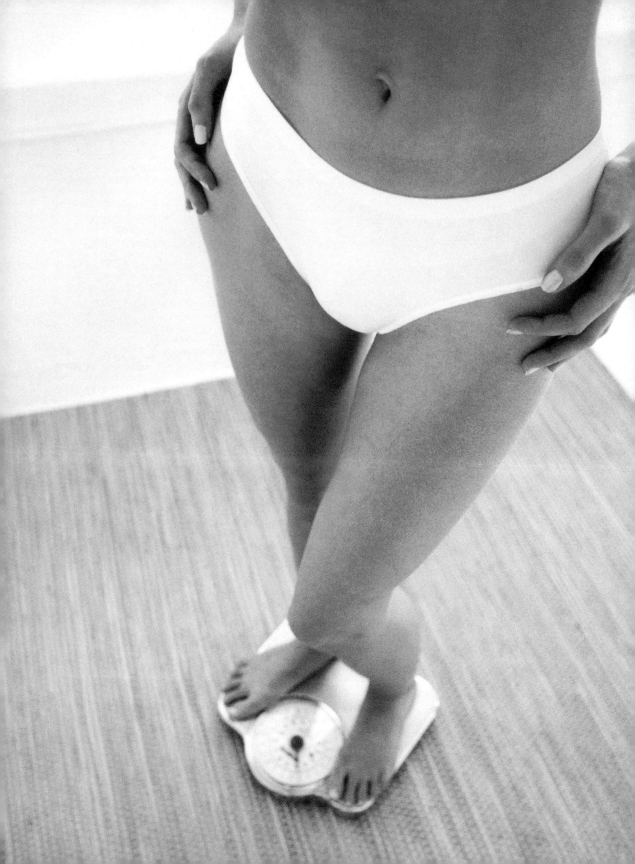

A good butt is dependant upon having a workable bodyweight. You cannot have a nicely rounded backside if you are too skinny or too overweight. If you are currently at either end of the scale you have to take action now. This cannot be accomplished just by taking in more or fewer calories. The exercise part of the equation must go hand in hand with eating the right foods. Healthy weight cannot be added or subtracted unless the food consumed is clean nutrition.

the skinny person's dilemma

Being underweight in our western world is not as big a problem as it once was. However, the underweight population in North America still runs into the millions. The quickest way to normalize a skinny person's body is to increase the ingestion of clean food: increase the number of meals per day and adopt a regular system of sensible weight training. Solid, healthy weight can come faster than you may imagine. Clean eating is the eating of good wholesome foods that have not been ruined by human intervention. When man has had his hand in the manufacture or packaging of a food, it usually ends up in the junk-food category. Clean-eating nutrition that comes to mind includes oatmeal, egg whites, poultry, fish, fruits, vegetables, whole grains, lean meats and salads.

Eat five to six small meals a day containing complex carbs (whole grains, nuts, rice, potatoes) and a high-protein food (skinless chicken breast, fish, egg whites). A high-quality protein drink supplement could be taken before retiring at night if you feel you need extra nutrition. Your weight-training schedule can be performed over two or three workouts a week. Once you have learned the simple exercises, a training session should never take longer than half an hour.

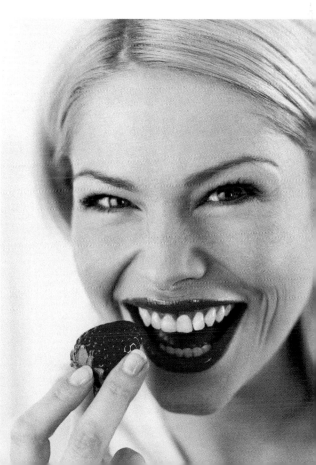

the overweight dilemma

A full 65 percent of North Americans are overweight. You can't have a great butt if you are overweight. Fat destroys shape.

Ironically, the way to lose weight is the same as to gain weight. We need to eat five or six times a day, smaller meals of course, but in many cases you will be eating more food than you have before. You won't be eating fat-, salt- and sugar-loaded foods like candies, cookies, cakes, doughnuts, chocolate, cereals and pies. Dairy products such as butter, margarine, lard, whole eggs, bacon, sausage, whole milk and cheese are not advised.

Excessively overweight people, those over 40, heavy smokers, or those who haven't exercised regularly should see their doctor and ask for a complete physical, including a stress test. Chances are your doctor will be thrilled at your proposed lifestyle adjustment and you will be given the go-ahead to change your eating and exercise habits. However, never neglect to consult your physician before starting any new diet or exercise regimen.

Exercise can be as mild as walking short stretches, increasing the pace or distance

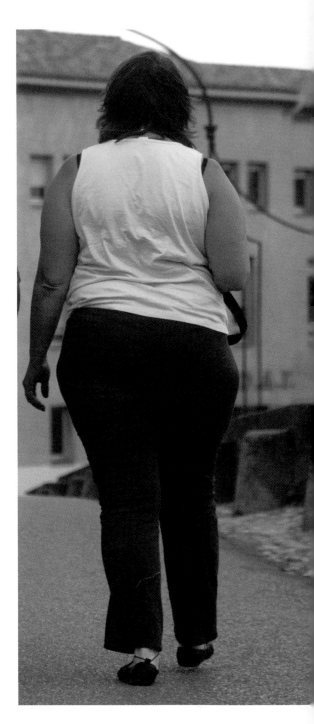

covered gradually, or as intense as full-fledged cardio activity. Always bear in mind that any new physical activity should be commenced with low duration and intensity. As time passes, both can be increased as your health and fitness levels improve.

Now listen to this: For years the U.S. and Canadian government agencies pushed the fact that weight control was a matter of calories-in-calories-out, also known as the bucket theory. This hypothesis says that the human body is like a bucket: the food you put in fills the bucket, and the exercise you do empties the bucket. So people who gain weight are just overfilling and under-emptying their buckets. The message is that we are all overeating and under-exercising. While that may be true, there is so much more to it than that. This bucket theory assumes that all calories can be treated equally, that all have the same impact on health and obesity. It neglects to take into account that foods vary hugely, not just in the amount of calories they produce, but in the way

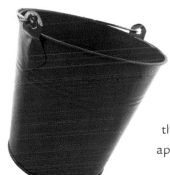

> The bucket theory assumes that all calories can be treated equally, that all have the same impact on health and obesity.

they contribute to the weight, health and appearance of the body.

The bucket theory is garbage. None of us should overeat, but it's not just the amount that is important. It's the dastardly trans fats, sugar and salt that give us the problem. Our cells are no longer able to function properly. It's the corruption of the food supply. And this is the reason to eat clean for the rest of your life. For more detailed information on clean eating, with lots of great tips and recipes, pick up a copy of my nutrition book: *The Eat-Clean Diet*.

eleven

butt
insights

Over the past ten months I have actively tried to dig deeper into the present butt culture. I needed to find out more about butt training: the little-known facts, the secrets from the mouths of the women with the best backsides in the world. The more I dug, the more I discovered. Here are a few more insights. Use them now or store them in your head for future use.

the 45° leg press

Leg-machine presses are found in most big gyms. They are seldom found in private homes. One of the best brands I know, and one I use regularly, is the Cybex machine. It's kind to the knees. With all the various butt exercises, why do we need yet another one? Answer: We don't need it. However, it's nice to have choices. If you have access to a 45° leg press machine, why not use it now and again? Variety is the spice of exercise success. The leg-press apparatus works the lower butt, right where you have a fold-over crease. Of course if you're very young right now you may not even have a crease but it's 10 to 1 you do, and 50 to 1 you do if you are over 20.

To get full "butt-action" from the leg press, bring the legs back to virtually touch the chest. Do not perform fast reps – no bouncing out of the bent-leg position. Lower the weight under control (fairly slowly). As your knees come to your chest you will notice your butt lifting off the backboard. This is the magic moment when the lower buttocks are worked. After three or four sets of 12 reps you will feel it in the tush – and what a great feeling!

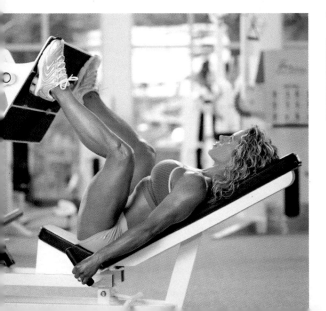

45° leg press

sets: 3-4
reps: 12

the adductor machine

This is another apparatus found only in big gyms or gyms with a comprehensive range of workable exercise apparatus. The adductor machine works the upper-inner thighs and the lateral glute area. Perform three sets of 15 reps at a moderate speed. You will feel the exercise more in your upper, inner thighs but believe me, the glutes are getting quite a workout too. If you haven't performed this exercise before, start light. After a few workouts you should begin piling on the resistance.

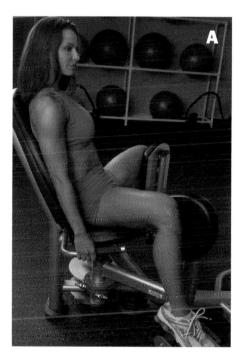

hip adductor

sets: 3
reps: 15

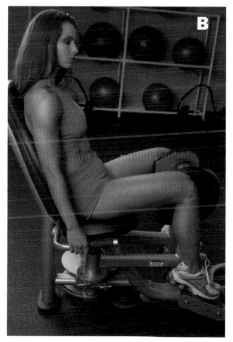

spinning

Many spinning classes are very rugged. Groups of individuals take positions on stationary bikes and pedal their way to fitness. Not only does spinning work the glutes, but calories are burned at a high rate.

Glutes are maximally worked when the bike rider is in a standing position as opposed to pedaling while seated. Naturally, the same effect can be obtained riding a regular bike, compounded by pedaling uphill in the standing position.

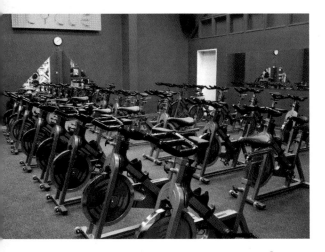

stair climbing

Advanced gym setups are not needed. They are convenient, yes, but not needed. Ironically, we will drive to the gym instead of making it on foot, only to go on a treadmill when we get there. We will ride an elevator instead of the stairs to take our place on a stepper. It doesn't line up with common sense, does it?

Climbing stairs to your office is a great way to train the butt. If you work or live on the 30th floor you may want to start more modestly, say take the stairs for ten floors and ride the elevator for twenty. Those already in super shape can do all thirty flights of stairs. Hey, if you're up for it, try two stairs at a time! Then you'll really get a butt workout! (A word of caution: please make sure your stairwell is safe, and use the buddy system.)

got access to a trampoline?

The other day I attended my daughter's gymnastics demonstration. One of the demonstrations was given by "older" members – people 40 years and up. One lady was in her late 60s and one gentleman had just celebrated his 71st birthday. What did I learn? That regular trampoline practice was extremely beneficial to the butt. These oldsters all had firm, rounded derrieres. It makes sense. Liftoff from the trampoline surface takes intense butt involvement and the return power-jolts the butt in such a unique way that the glute muscles are hugely involved. Presto! More tone, rotundity and overall appeal. I know if you put these tips to good use you will be taking giant steps toward the butt you've always wanted.

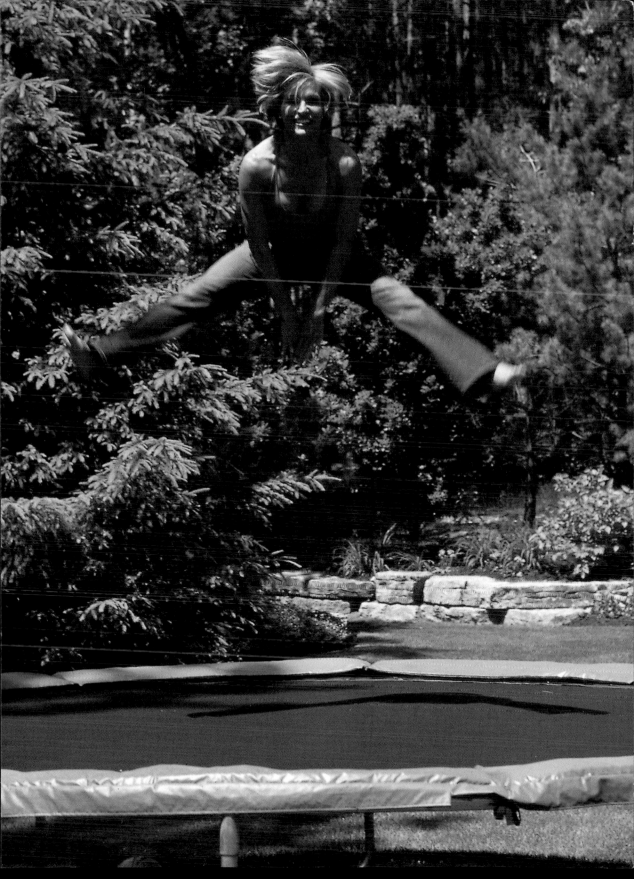

A

Abdominals – The series of muscles located on the lower midsection of the torso. They are used to contract the body forward through a range of six to eight inches.

Aerobic Exercise – Any long-lasting exercise that can be carried on within the body's ability to replenish oxygen in working muscles.

AIDS – Short for Acquired Immune Deficiency Syndrome. AIDS is caused by a virus and is contracted by the exchange of bodily fluids. There have been some cases of bodybuilders contracting AIDS from the sharing of needles (used for anabolic steroid injections).

Amenorrhea – Absence of menstrual periods often caused by low body-fat percentage.

Amino Acids – Called the "building blocks of life," amino acids are biochemical subunits linked together by chemical bonds to form polypeptide chains. Hundreds of polypeptides, in turn, link together to form a protein molecule.

Anabolic – Metabolic process whereby smaller units are assembled into larger units. For example, the combining of amino acids into protein strands is a form of anabolism.

Anaerobic Exercise – Any high-intensity exercise that outstrips the body's aerobic capacity and leads to an oxygen debt. Because of its intensity, anaerobic exercise can be maintained for only short periods of time.

Arthritis – Chronic condition marked by an inflammation of the tissue surrounding the joints.

Asymmetric Training – Any exercise that targets only one side of the body. One-arm dumbell curls, lateral raises and one-arm triceps extensions are all examples of asymmetric training.

B

Back – The series of muscles located on the dorsal region of the body. The back muscle complex includes the latissimus dorsi, spinal erectors, trapezius, rhomboids and teres minor and major.

Barbell – One of the most basic pieces of bodybuilding equipment. Barbells consist of a long bar, collars, sleeves, and associated plates made of steel or iron. They may be either adjustable (allowing the changing of plates) or fixed (the plates are kept in place by welded collars). Barbells average between five and seven feet in length, and usually weigh between 25 and 45 pounds.

Basic Exercises – Exercises that work more than one muscle group simultaneously. Basic exercises form the mainstay of a bodybuilder's mass-gaining routine. Examples include: bench presses, shoulder presses, squats, deadlifts, and bent-over rows.

Belt – Large leather support worn around the waist by bodybuilders. Weightlifting belts are usually four to six inches in width and provide support to the lower-back muscles and spine.

Biceps – Flexor muscles located on the upper arm. The biceps are composed of two "heads," and are responsible for bending the lower arm towards the upper arm.

Biofeedback – Any physiological or psychological symptom given off by the body. The best bodybuilders are those who recognize such biofeedback signals and use them to improve their training, eating, and competitive preparation.

BMR – Short for Basil Metabolic Rate, the BMR is the speed at which the resting body consumes energy (calories).

Body-fat Percentage – The ratio of fat to bodyweight. For most women, seventeen to twenty percent is ideal.

Breathing Pullovers – Specialized exercise important to a bodybuilder as it stretches the rib cartilage, producing a large rib cage and, therefore, a larger chest measurement.

Burn – Term unique to physique training, describing the feeling a muscle gets as it's exercised. Burns are partial reps done at the end of a set when performing full reps is impossible.

Bursae – Flat sacks filled with fluid. They support and protect joints.

Buttocks – Another term referring to the gluteus maximus, medius and minimus, extensors and abductors of the thigh at the hip joint.

C

Cables – Long wire cords attached to weight stacks at one end and a hand grip at the other. Cable exercises keep tension on the working muscle throughout a full range of motion.

Calves – Also called "lowers" and "bodybuilding's diamonds," the calves consist of the soleus and gastrocnemius muscles located on the backs of the lower leg bones. The calves are similar to the forearms in that they are composed of extremely dense muscle tissue. Their function is to extend the ankles.

Carbohydrate Loading – The practice of depleting and replenishing the body's glycogen levels in the weeks leading up to a bodybuilding contest. This technique allows bodybuilders to saturate their muscles with stored water, thus making the muscles fuller and harder.

Cartilage – Connective tissue that acts as a shock absorber between bones. It's found wherever two bones articulate over one another.

Cheating – An advanced training technique that consists of utilizing fresh muscles to assist in the completion of an exercise, when the muscle being trained is nearing fatigue.

Chelation – The process by which protein molecules are bonded to inorganic minerals, making them easier to assimilate by the human body.

Chest – The large pectoral muscles located on the front of the upper torso, responsible for drawing the arms toward the center of the body.

Cholesterol – Naturally occurring steroid molecule involved in the formation of hormones, vitamins, bile salts and the transport of fats in the bloodstream to tissues throughout the body. Excessive cholesterol in the diet can lead to cardiovascular disease.

Circuit Training – A specialized form of weight training that combines strength training and aerobic conditioning. Circuit training consists of performing 10 to 20 different exercises, one after the other, with little rest between sets.

Collar – Small round iron or plastic clamp, used to anchor plates on a barbell or dumbell. In most cases collars are screwed on but some versions are held in a spring-like manner.

Compound Exercises – Any exercise that works more than one muscle group. Popular compound movements include: bench presses, squats, shoulder presses, and bent-over rows.

Cortisol – Catabolic hormone released by the body in response to stress (of which exercise is one form). Cortisol speeds up the rate at which large units are broken down into smaller units (catabolism).

Cut – Competitive term used to describe the physical appearance of a physique competitor. To be "cut" implies that you are in great competitive shape, with extremely low body-fat levels.

Cycle Training – Form of training where high-intensity workouts are alternated with those of low intensity. The technique can be applied weekly or yearly.

D

Decline Bench – Bench used to work the lower and outer pectorals. Decline benches require the user to place their head at the low end and their feet at the upper end of the bench.

Definition – Another term to describe the percentage of body-fat carried by a competitive bodybuilder. A bodybuilder with good definition shows a great deal of vascularity and muscle separation.

Dehydration Biological state where the body has insufficient water levels for proper functioning. As the human body is over 90 percent water, athletes must continuously replenish the water lost during intense exercise.

Density – Term used to describe the amount of muscle mass carried by a bodybuilder. It generally refers to muscle thickness and hardness.

Descending Sets – An advanced training technique involving the removal of weight at the completion of a set, and then the performing of additional reps with the lighter weight.

Diet – A term that refers to a fixed eating pattern. In general usage it usually means to try and lose weight.

Dislocation – Type of injury where the end of one bone (called a "ball") slips out of a hollow indentation (called the "socket") of another bone. It is usually accompanied by tearing of the joint ligaments, which makes the injury extremely painful.

Diuretics – Some bodybuilders use diuretics before a contest as it improves their muscularity. Diuretics are any natural or synthetic chemical that causes the body to excrete water. In most cases the drug interacts with aldosterone, the hormone responsible for water retention. Diuretics also flush electrolytes from the body. One of the functions of electrolytes is to control heart rate, so using diuretics to get "cut" is a dangerous practice. A few pro bodybuilders have died of diuretic-induced heart attacks.

Down the Rack – An advanced training technique involving the use of two or three successively lighter dumbells during the performance of one set.

Dumbell – Short bars on which plates are secured. Dumbells can be considered the one-arm version of a barbell. In most gyms, the weight plates are welded on, and the poundage is written on the dumbell.

E

Ectomorphs – Body type characterized by long thin bones, low body-fat levels, and difficulty in gaining muscle mass.

Endomorphs – Body type characterized by large bones and an excess of body-fat.

Endorphins – Chemicals released by the brain in response to pain. Often called "natural opiates," endorphins decrease the individual's sensitivity to pain.

Exercise – In general terms, any form of physical activity that increases the heart and respiratory rate. In bodybuilding terms, an exercise is one specific movement for one or more muscle groups.

EZ-curl Bar – Short, S-shaped bar used for such exercises as biceps curls and lying triceps extensions. The bar's unique shape puts less stress on the wrists and forearms than a straight bar.

F

Flexibility – The degree of muscle and connective tissue suppleness at a joint. The greater the flexibility, the greater the range of movement by an individual's limbs and torso.

Fast-twitch Muscle Fiber – Type of muscle fiber that is adapted for rapid but short duration contractions.

Fluid Retention – Bodybuilding term referring to the amount of water held between the skin and muscles. A bodybuilder "holding water" appears smooth, and his muscularity is blurred.

Forced Reps – An advanced training technique where a training partner helps you complete extra reps after the exercised muscles reach the point of fatigue.

Fracture – Complete or partial break of one of the body's bones.

Free Weights – Term given to barbells and dumbells. Free-weight exercises are the most popular types performed by bodybuilders.

G

Genetics – The study of how biological traits or characteristics are passed from one generation to the next. In physique building terms it refers to the potential each individual has for developing his or her physique.

Giant Sets – An advanced training technique wherein four or more exercises are performed consecutively. In most cases the term refers to exercises for one muscle group, but bodybuilders have been known to use exercises for four different muscle groups.

Gloves – Specialized hand apparel worn while working out. Gloves help prevent blisters and calluses.

Glycogen – Primary fuel source used by exercising muscles. Glycogen is one of the stored forms of carbohydrate.

Golgi Tendon Organ (GTI) – Stretch receptors located at the ends of muscles. They terminate muscular contractions when too much stress is placed on the muscle.

Gym – Although this can apply to almost any exercising venue (e.g. high school gym), for bodybuilders the term refers to a weight-training club.

H

Hamstrings – The leg biceps located on the back of the upper legs, responsible for curling the lower leg toward the upper leg. The hamstrings are analogous to the biceps in the upper arm.

Head Straps – Leather or nylon harness that is placed over the head, allowing the user to attach weight and train the neck muscles.

Hypertrophy – Biological term that means muscle growth. Muscles do not grow by increasing the number of cells, but rather by increasing the size of existing muscle fibers.

I

Injuries – Physical injuries include any damage to bone, muscle, or connective tissue. The most common bodybuilding injuries are muscle strains.

Instinctive Training – An advanced training technique whereby one trains according to how he or she "feels." In short, you deviate from the normal routine and train according to intuition. It takes many years of experience to become in tune enough with your body to train instinctively.

Intercostals – Small, finger-like muscles located along the sides of the lower abdomen, between the rib cage and the obliques.

Isolation Exercises – Any exercise aimed at working only one muscle. In most cases, it's virtually impossible to totally isolate a muscle. Some common examples are: preacher curls, lateral raises, and triceps pushdowns.

Isometric – Type of muscle contraction in which there is no shortening of the muscle's length. Isometric exercises were popularized by Charles Atlas.

Isotension – Exercising technique wherein continuous stress is placed on a given muscle. Extending the leg by contracting the quadriceps, and holding the position for 10 to 20 seconds or more, is an example of isotension. Bodybuilders make use of the technique during the precompetition phase as it improves muscle separation.

Isotonic – Type of muscle contraction wherein the contracting muscle shortens. The muscle may also be lengthening, as when doing a "negative." Most resistance exercises are examples of isotonic contraction.

J

Joint – The point at which two bones meet. Most joints have a hinge-type structure that allows the bones to articulate (bend) over one another.

L

Lactic Acid – A product given off during aerobic respiration. Lactic acid was once thought to be strictly a waste product, however, recent evidence suggests that a version of lactic acid called lactate is used by the liver to replenish glycogen supplies.

Latissimus Dorsi – Called the lats, these large fan-shaped muscles are located on the back of the torso, and when properly developed give the bodybuilder the characteristic V-shape. The lats function to pull the arms down and back.

Layoff – Any extended time spent away from the gym is called a layoff. It can be referred to as a training vacation.

Ligament – Fibrous connective tissue that joins one bone to another.

M

Massage – Recovery technique that involves a forceful rubbing, pinching, or kneading, of the body's muscles. Massage speeds up the removal rate of exercise byproducts, helps athletes relax, and improves performance. The most popular forms of massage are Soviet and Swedish.

Mesomorphs – Body type characterized by large bones, low body-fat levels, and a greater-than-average rate of muscle growth.

Muscularity – Another term used to describe the degree of muscular definition. The lower the body-fat percentage the greater the degree of muscularity.

Muscle – The series of tissue bellies located on the skeleton that serve to move and stabilize the body's various appendages.

N

Negatives – A portion of the rep movement that goes in the same direction as gravity. The trainer concentrates on resisting the movement.

Neuromuscular System – The combination of nerves and muscles that interact to control body movement.

Nutrition – The art of combining foods in the right amounts so the human body receives all of the required nutrients. In bodybuilding terms, eating to gain muscle size and reduce body-fat levels is considered proper nutrition.

Nutrients – The various minerals, vitamins, proteins, fats, and carbohydrates needed by the body for proper maintenance, health, and growth.

O

Oil – Mineral or water-based liquid used by physique competitors to highlight the muscles while onstage. Most use vegetable oils as they are absorbed by the skin and give it a better texture.

Olympic Barbell – The most specialized and refined barbell in weightlifting. Olympic barbells weigh 45 pounds and are made from spring-steel.

Overload – Term used to describe the degree of stress placed on a muscle. To overload means to continuously increase the amount of resistance that a muscle has to work against. For bodybuilders the stress is in the form of weight.

Overtraining – The physiological state whereby the individual's recovery system is taxed to the limit. In many cases, insufficient time is allowed for recovery between workouts. Among the more common symptoms are: muscle loss, lack of motivation, insomnia, and reduced energy.

P

Peak – This can mean the degree of sharpness or shape held by a particular muscle (usually the biceps), or it may refer to the shape a bodybuilder or fitness competitor holds on a given contest day. A woman who has "peaked" is in top condition.

Plateau – A state of training where no progress is being made. Plateaus usually occur after long periods of repetitious training. Breaking the condition involves shocking the muscles with new training techniques.

Plates – Small to large cast-iron weights that are placed on a barbell or dumbell. Plates range in size from 1 1/4 pounds to 100 pounds. The most common plates in bodybuilding gyms weigh 5, 10, 25, 35, and 45 pounds.

Posing – The art of displaying the physique in a bodybuilding or fitness contest.

Positives – Part of the rep movement that goes against gravity. In barbell biceps curls, the positive phase would occur during the curling of the barbell. The lowering of the bar is the negative phase.

Poundage – Another term used to describe the weight of a barbell, dumbell, or machine weight stack.

Pre-exhaust – Advanced training technique first described by *MuscleMag's* Robert Kennedy. The technique involves fatiguing a desired muscle with an isolation movement, and then using a compound exercise to stress the muscle even further. Pre-exhaust is ideal for eliminating the "weakest link in the chain" effect often encountered during compound exercises.

Priority Training – Training strategy where an individual devotes most of her energy to targeting weak muscle groups.

Proportion – Term used to describe the size of one muscle with respect to the whole body. A bodybuilder or fitness competitor with good "proportions" would have all her muscles in balance with regards to muscle size.

Protein – Nutrient composed of long chains of amino acids. Protein is primarily used in the production of muscle tissue, hormones, and enzymes.

Pump – Biological condition where an exercised muscle swells and becomes engorged with blood.

Pumping Up – The practice of performing light exercise just before walking onstage at a contest. Pumping up gives the muscles a temporary size increase.

Pyramiding – Training technique in which weight is added for the first couple of sets and then decreased for the remaining sets. A half pyramid technique may also be performed, where the weight is only added or only decreased for the given number of sets.

Q

Quadriceps – Commonly known as the "thighs," the quads are the large, four-headed muscles located on the front and sides of the upper legs. They are analogous to the triceps, and are the extensors of the legs. Their primary function is to extend the knee, bringing the lower leg forward (bringing the upper and lower legs to a locked-out configuration).

R

Repetition – Abbreviated "rep," this simply refers to one full movement of a particular exercise.

Resistance – The amount of force being placed on a muscle. In bodybuilding circles it refers to the amount of weight being lifted.

Rest/Pause – A training technique where the user completes one set, and then rests about 10 seconds before starting the next set. The technique is based on the biological fact that a muscle recovers about 90 percent of its strength within 10 to 15 seconds.

Ripped – Another term to describe the percentage of body fat carried by a competitive bodybuilder. A ripped bodybuilder has a very low body-fat percentage (eight to twelve percent).

Routine – Another word for program, schedule, agenda, etc. It refers to the complete number of sets, reps, and exercises performed for a given muscle or muscles on a particular day.

S

Set – Term referring to a given number of consecutive reps. For example, 10 nonstop reps would be called one "set" of 10.

Shocking – Training strategy that involves training the muscle with a new form of exercise. Shocking techniques are used to "kick start" muscles that have become accustomed to repetitious training routines.

Shoulders – The deltoid muscles – anterior, medial and posterior – located at the top of the torso. The deltoids are responsible for elevating and rotating the shoulder girdle.

Sleeve – Short, hollow, metal tube fitted over both ends of a barbell. The sleeve allows the plates to rotate on the bar, thus reducing the stress on the user's wrists.

Slow-twitch Muscle Fiber – Type of muscle fiber adapted for slow, long duration contraction. The spinal erectors of the lower back are primarily composed of slow-twitch muscle fibers.

Somatotype – Term referring to an individual's body characteristics, including such things as muscle size, bone size, body-fat level, and personality.

Soreness – The mild pain felt in muscles after a workout. It is primarily caused by lactic acid build-up, and usually appears 12 to 24 hours after exercising.

Spinal Erectors – Two long, snake-like muscles located at the center of the lower back. The spinal erectors help maintain posture by keeping the upper body perpendicular with the floor.

Split Routines – Any routine in which different muscle groups are worked on separate days. The most common split routines are four- and six-day splits.

Spot – In short, a helping hand when performing a particular exercise. A spot is provided by a training partner when you fail during an exercise. In most cases it involves providing a few pounds of upward pressure to keep the barbell, dumbell, or machine handle moving.

Staggered Sets – An advanced training technique where the user adds sets for a weak muscle group between sets of her regular training exercises. For example, many bodybuilders with weak calves add extra calf training between sets for other muscle groups. In many cases, the calf exercise is performed instead of taking a rest.

Steroids – Synthetic derivatives of the hormone testosterone that allow the user to gain muscle mass and strength more rapidly.

Sticking Point – The point during an exercise where the user is in the weakest biomechanical position. In other words, this is the most difficult part of the movement. The sticking point is usually close to the bottom of an exercise.

Straps – Long, narrow pieces of material used to increase one's gripping power on an exercise. Straps are wrapped around the lower forearm and bar in such a manner that as the user grips the bar, the straps get tighter. They are used on such exercises as deadlifts, shrugs, and chins.

Stretching – Form of exercise for which the primary goal is to increase flexibility. Stretching is also an excellent way to warm up the body and prepare it for more stressful forms of exercise.

Stretch Marks – Red or purple lines caused by thinning and loss of elasticity in the skin.

Strict Form – Training technique that involves performing exercises in a slow, controlled manner, and through a full range of motion, without the aid of a partner or cheating techniques.

Stripping Method – An advanced training technique wherein the individual removes a few plates at the end of a set and forces out extra reps. The technique allows the user to force a muscle past the point of normal failure.

Supersets – Advanced training technique wherein two exercises are performed consecutively without any rest. Supersets may consist of exercises for the same muscle group (e.g. dumbell curls and barbell curls) or exercises for different muscle groups (e.g. triceps extensions and biceps curls). When performing supersets for different muscle groups, it is common to work opposing muscle groups (triceps/biceps, quads/hamstrings, chest/back, etc.).

Supination – Technique in which an appendage rolls away from the midpoint of the body. For example, the palms start off facing the body during a dumbell curl, and rotate outward as the dumbell is raised. At the top of the movement, the palms are facing upward. The technique takes advantage of the wrist-rotating properties of the biceps.

Supplements – Any form of vitamin, mineral, protein or other nutrient that is taken separately from, or in addition to, normal food. Supplements come in many forms including tablet, capsule, powder, oil, or plant material.

Sweat Bands – Small pieces of material, usually cloth, wrapped around the forehead to absorb sweat.

Symmetry – Symmetry means right-left balance. In bodybuilding this term often refers to the overall balance of the body. Symmetry is closely related to proportion. A bodybuilder with good symmetry does not have any overdeveloped or underdeveloped muscle groups.

T

Tanning – Biochemical reaction where the skin releases pigment upon exposure to sunlight (or artificial tanning light). Competitors tan because a darker complexion improves skin's appearance in a contest or photoshoot, highlighting muscularity.

Tendinitis – Form of inflammation involving tendons and the points where they attach to muscles and bones. Tendinitis is usually caused by overstressing a particular area. Bodybuilders often get tendinitis in the biceps-tendon region.

Tendon – Tough cord of connective tissue that joins a muscle to a bone.

Testosterone – Androgenic/anabolic hormone responsible for such physiological effects as: increasing muscle size and strength, facial hair growth, scalp hair loss, sperm production (males), and increasing aggression levels. Although both sexes have circulating testosterone, males have it in greater concentrations.

Training Diary – Daily journal, or record, useful for keeping track of such items as weight, exercises, sets, reps, calories and overall motivation levels.

Training Partner – Any individual who matches you set for set during your workout. Training partners allow you to go for that extra rep and act as spotters. They also serve as a sort of coach on days when you just don't feel like working out.

Training to Failure – Any time you terminate a set only after the muscle cannot contract for an additional rep. Most bodybuilders train to positive failure and then have a training partner help them perform a few extra reps – but not on every set.

Triceps – Extensor muscles of the upper arm. The triceps are composed of three "heads," and work in opposition to the biceps in that they extend the lower arm to a locked-out position.

Trisets – Similar to supersets but involving the use of three different exercises for the same muscle group.

Twenty-ones – Advanced exercise technique in which you perform seven half-reps of a given exercise at the bottom of the movement, seven half-reps at the top, and finish with seven full reps.

U

Universal Machine – The most common type of training apparatus (not counting free weights) found in bodybuilding gyms. The machines may train one muscle group or may have numerous stations to train the whole body.

V

Vascularity – The degree of vein and artery visibility. In order to be "highly" vascular, a bodybuilder must have an extremely low body-fat percentage.

Warmup – Any form of light, short duration exercise that prepares the body for more intense exercise. Warming up should involve increasing the heart and respiratory rate, and stretching. A good warmup helps prevent injury.

W

Weight – This term refers to the plates or weight stacks themselves, or it can be used to describe the actual poundage on the bar.

Weightlifting – A term used to describe weight training, or an Olympic event. The competitive version involves two lifts – the snatch, and the clean and jerk.

Workout – The program or schedule of exercises performed on any given day.

Wraps – Long pieces of material (usually a first-aid bandage) that bodybuilders wrap around weak or injured bodyparts. Wraps keep the area warm and provide extra security. Many bodybuilders wrap the knees during squats, and the wrists during bench presses.

credits

FRONT/BACK COVER PHOTO CREDIT:
Robert Reiff

INTERIOR PHOTO CREDITS:
Alex Ardenti: page 31, 112

Brahm Verhoeckx: page 53 (garlic herbed fish), 59 & 77 (fillet of sole), 89

Robert Reiff: page 5, 6, 9, 17, 28, 50 (meals & soup), 51 (meals), 52 (meals), 53 & 66 (Swiss Muesli), 54 (meals & soup), 55 (meals), 56 (meals & soup), 57 (meals), 58 (meals), 59 (meals), 60 (meals & soup), 61(meals), 62 (meals & soup), 63 (all meals), 70, 73, 81, 82, 92, 99, 100, 103, 104, 106, 110 (photo of butt),116, 117 (plate), 120 (model), 134

Cathy Chatterton: page 30, 39, 47, 114

Cory Sorensen: page 21, 45 (dinner dish), 48, 55 (baked salmon), 58 (Curried Pumpkin Soup), 61 (Seared Tuna), 69, 74, 78, 85, 117

fotolia: page 40, 41, 43 (butter), 44 (fish dish), 45 (yogurt), 52 & 95 & 96 (soup), 76, 90, 109 (butt), 110 (fridge), 118, 120 (cellulite), 121, 120, 126, 127, 131 (bucket), 132, 136

istockphoto: page 10, 11, 27, 38, 44 (green tea & vitamins), 45 (water bottles), 64, 109 (junk food), 111, 115, 130

Lisa Bouvier Brewer: page135

Sebastian Cimetta: page 18

Terry Goodlad: page 3, 108

Robert Kennedy: page 137

ILLUSTRATION CREDITS:
Stephanie Bratt: page 14, 15

Ted Hammond: page 22, 23, 24, 25, 26, 32, 33, 34, 35, 36, 37